Medical Finals:

Short cases with structured answers

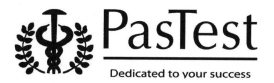

PasTest

Dedicated to your success

Medical Finals:

Short cases with structured answers

Second edition

Adam Feather MB MRCP
Consultant in Medicine for the Elderly
Newham University Hospital Trust, London

Benjamin C.T. Field MBBS BMedSci MSc MRCP
MRC Clinical Research Training Fellow,
Imperial College London
Hammersmith Hospital, London

Ramanathan Visvanathan BM FRCS
Consultant surgeon, Bronglais General Hospital, Aberystwyth
Honorary Lecturer, University of Wales College of Medicine
Surgical Tutor, Royal College of Surgeons of England
Lately Honorary Senior Lecturer and Assistant Director,
Professorial Surgical Unit, St. Bartholomew's Hospital, London

John S P Lumley MS FRCS
Emeritus Professor of Vascular Surgery, St. Bartholomew's and the Royal
London School of Medicine and Dentistry
Honorary Consultant Surgeon,
St. Bartholomew's Hospital, London
Member of Council, Royal College of Surgeons and England,
Past World President, International College of Surgeons

© 2007 PASTEST LTD
Egerton Court
Parkgate Estate
Knutsford
Cheshire
WA16 8DX

Telephone: 01565 752000

First Published 1997
Second edition 2007

ISBN: 1 905635 10 9
ISBN: 978 1 905635 108

A catalogue record for this book is available from the British Library.

The information contained within this book was obtained by the author from reliable sources. However, while every effort has been made to ensure its accuracy, no responsibility for loss, damage or injury occasioned to any person acting or refraining from action as a result of information contained herein can be accepted by the publishers or author.

PasTest Revision Books and Intensive Courses

PasTest has been established in the field of postgraduate medical education since 1972, providing revision books and intensive study courses for doctors preparing for their professional examinations.

Books and courses are available for the following specialties:
MRCGP, MRCP Parts 1 and 2, MRCPCH Parts 1 and 2, MRCPsych, MRCS, MRCOG Parts 1 and 2, DRCOG, DCH, FRCA, PLAB Parts 1 and 2.

For further details contact:
**PasTest, Freepost, Knutsford, Cheshire WA16 7BR
Tel: 01565 752000   Fax: 01565 650264
www.pastest.co.uk   enquiries@pastest.co.uk**

Text prepared by Saxon Graphics Ltd, Derby
Printed and bound in the UK by Athenaeum Press, Gateshead

Contents

Preface

Our collaboration ten years ago for the first edition of this book produced a volume at the forefront of medical undergraduate assessment. Many things have changed since then and this new edition has tried to place itself yet again as a leader, rather than a follower, of present and future trends in this area. Many UK, North American and European medical schools have adopted assessment formats that can either be completed on and / or marked by computer software. Unfortunately, the software is still unable to recognise free text and so is limited in its application. EMQs and MCQs remain the predominant methods of undergraduate assessment in many countries in the world. However, it is obvious to us that 'free response' answers, far from being defunct, will once again become 'assessment de jour' once the software catches up – surely just a few years away. Short answer questions (SAQs) are an extremely important method of assessment at all levels of the undergraduate and postgraduate programme and have many important facets that are lacking with other assessment formats.

SAQs are used to test clinical problem solving, reasoning and management as well as ethico-legal and multidisciplinary aspects of a case. They are easier for students to complete, allowing them good insight into the marking scheme and the important areas within each question. SAQs still need to be marked by examiners, but with clear marking guides and simple, clear structuring they remain far easier to review than the traditional essay.

This edition retains the majority of previous questions, covering the most frequently tested and clinically relevant topics to students in the latter phases of their course. However, we have made some welcome additions to each chapter and all the answers have been updated, to include the latest management and clinical thinking. The previous use of answer boxes has been dropped in order to incorporate the new and elaborated questions and answers.

Although this book is not intended as a comprehensive text, the range of questions provides a broad base for revision purposes. It may also be used as a learning aid, together with medical texts and other information sources, and we have included many web links at the end of the expanded answer sections. Whatever method of assessment is presently in vogue, the text provides the reader with a useful and challenging method of self-assessment, enabling the reader to check his or her progress towards graduation.

Acknowledgements
We wish to thank our families for their support and understanding, Amy Thornton and Cathy Dickens, our publishers, for their patience and support in the production of this new edition.

Revision checklist

Chapter 1: Infection
Streptococcal and staphyloccoccal infections
Atypical pneumonias
Tuberculosis
Meningitis
Viral hepatitis
HIV and associated diseases
Sexually transmissable diseases
Malaria
Parasitic infection

Chapter 2: Metabolic Diseases
Wilson's disease
Haemochromatosis
Porphyria
Hyperlipidaemia
Rickets/osteomalacia

Chapter 3: Neurology
Strokes – including subarachnoid haemorrhage
Epilepsy
Multiple sclerosis
Parkinson's disease
Space occupying lesions
Cranial nerve lesions
Peripheral neuropathy
Cerebellar lesions
Myasthenia gravis
Motor neurone disease

Chapter 4: Endocrinology
Diabetes mellitus
Thyrotoxicosis and hypothyroidism
Hypothalamic–pituitary–gonadal axis
Acromegaly
Cushing's syndrome and Addison's disease
Hypercalcaemia
Secondary causes of hypertension

Chapter 5: Respiratory Medicine
Pneumonia (bacterial and viral)
Asthma
Pulmonary tuberculosis
Chronic obstructive pulmonary disease
Bronchogenic carcinoma
Cystic fibrosis and bronchiectasis
Fibrotic lung diseases
Industrial lung diseases

Chapter 6: Cardiology
Ischaemic heart disease
Cardiac failure
Valvular heart disease
Arrhythmias
Endocarditis
Cardiomyopathy
Hypertension

Chapter 7: Haematology
Microcytic and macrocytic anaemia
Haemolytic anaemia
Aplastic anaemia
Leukaemia
Lymphoma
Myeloma
Thrombocytopenia
Bleeding disorders
Transfusion reactions

Chapter 8: Dermatology
Eczema
Psoriasis
Erythema multiforme
Dermatological manifestations of systemic disease
Skin malignancies
Nail disorders
Hair disorders

Chapter 9: Gastroenterology
Dysphagia
Peptic ulcer disease
Coeliac disease and malabsorptive states
Inflammatory bowel disease
Gastrointestinal bleeds
Viral hepatitis
Alcoholic liver disease
Autoimmune liver disease viii

Chapter 10: Nephrology
Urinary tract infection
Nephrotic syndrome
Glomerulonephritis
Acute and chronic renal failure
Diabetic nephropathy
Polycystic kidney disease
Secondary causes of hypertension

Chapter 11: Rheumatology and Connective Tissue Disease
Rheumatoid arthritis
Osteoarthritis
Systemic lupus erythematosus
Systemic sclerosis
Gout and pyrophosphate arthropathy
The systemic vasculitides – Wegener's granulomatosis and
polyarteritis nodosa
Reiter's syndrome
Septic arthritis
Osteoporosis

Chapter 12: Psychiatry
Schizophrenia
Depression
Mania
Personality disorder
Drug addiction and abuse
Alcohol abuse
Eating disorders

Chapter 13: Care of the Elderly
Falls
Dementia and confusional states
Mental incapacity legislation
Incontinence
Mobility problems
Terminal illness
The multidisciplinary team

Recommended reading list

Get a concensus – asking senior students, tutors, and foundation doctors should give you a good idea of the books to buy. A visit to your medical college bookshop should also give you a good guide particularly for newer textbooks.

Break the habit of a lifetime – visit the college library. This will allow you to choose the books that best suit you. Most good bookshops will also allow you to 'peruse' the shelves before making a commitment.

Make a personal choice – often choices of textbooks come down to personal views and finances. Buy the book that best suits you but also bear in mind a good textbook should last well into post-graduate years.

WWW – Many textbooks now have associated websites and are available on CD-ROM or equivalent. It is worth checking out the links that the books supply to see which are most easy to navigate and are most helpful to your learning approach. I would also recommend the website [**http: //www.emedicine.com/specialties.htm** which not only provides up-to-date reviews on most medical subjects but is well referenced and easy to use.

The following are all excellent medical textbooks which should be found in all good medical bookshops and the school library.

(1) Oxford Textbook of Medicine 4th Edition, July 2005. Edited by David A. Warrell et al. Oxford University Press

(2) Kumar and Clark Clinical Medicine – 6th Edition, August 2005; Edited by Parveen Kumar and Michael Clark. Elsevier

(3) Acute Clinical Medicine – 1st edition, 2005 Edited by Parveen Kumar and Michael Clark. Elsevier

(4) Textbook of Medicine, 4th Edition, 2003, Edited by Robert L Souhami and John Moxham

(5) Davidson's Principles and Practice of Medicine, 20th edition June 2006 Edited by Nicholas A. Boon et al. Churchill Livingstone

(6) Harrison's Principles of Internal Medicine 16th Edition, 2004 Edited by Kasper et al. McGraw-Hill Education

Abbreviations

5HT	5-hydroxytryptamine
AAFB	alcohol and acid fast bacilli
ABG	arterial blood gas
ACE	angiotensin-converting enzyme
ACE(I)	angiotensin-converting enzyme (inhibitor)
ACh	acetylcholine
ACTH	adrenocorticotrophic hormone
ADL	activities of daily living
AF	atrial fibrillation
AIDS	acquired immunodeficiency syndrome
ALL	acute lymphoblastic leukaemia
ALT	alanine aminotransferase
AML	acute myeloid leukaemia
ANCA	antineutrophil cytoplasmic antibody
ANF	antinuclear factor
ARDS	adult respiratory distress syndrome
ASO	antistreptolysin
AST	aspartate transaminase
AV	atrio-ventricular
AXR	abdominal X-ray abdominal radiograph
BCG	bacille Calmette–Guérin
bd	*bis in die* (twice a day)
BMI	body mass index
BP	blood pressure
C	centigrade
CAH	congenital adrenal hypoplasia
CAPD	continuous ambulatory peritoneal dialysis
CDH	congenital dislocation of the hip
CF	cystic fibrosis
CJD	Creutzfeldt–Jakob disease
CK-MB	creatine kinase-MB

CLL	chronic lymphoblastic leukaemia
cm	centimeter
CML	chronic myeloid leukaemia
CMV	cytomegalovirus
CNS	central nervous system
CPAP	continuous positive airways pressure
CPK	creatine phosphokinase
CRH	corticotrophin-releasing hormone
CSF	cerebrospinal fluid
CSU	catheter specimen of urine
CT	computed tomography
CTPA	computed tomography pulmonary angiogram
Cu	copper
CVA	cerebrovascular accident (stroke)
CVP	central venous pressure
CXR	chest X-ray
DDAVP	desmopressin
DEXA	dual-energy X-ray absorptiometry
DHEAS	dihydroepiandrosterone sulphate
DIC	disseminated intravascular coagulation
DMARD	disease-modifying agent of rheumatological disease
DSA	digital subtraction angio *or* arteriography
dsDNA	double-stranded DNA
DVT	deep vein thrombosis
EBV	Epstein–Barr virus
ECG	electrocardiography
ECT	electroconvulsive therapy
EEG	electroencephalography
EMG	electromyelography
EPO	erythropoietin
ESR	erythrocyte sedimentation rate
FBC	full blood count
FCV	forced vital capacity
FDG-PET	^{18}F-fluorodeoxyglucose positron emission tomography
FDP	fibrin *or* fibrinogen degradation products
Fe	iron
FEV	forced expiratory volume
FFP	fresh-frozen plasma

fl	femtolitre
FSH	follicle-stimulating hormone
FTA	fluorescent *Treponema* antibodies-absorbed test
g/dl	grams per decilitre
g/l	grams per litre
GABA	gamma-aminobutyric acid
GAD	glutamic acid decarboxylase
gamma GT	gamma-glutamyl transferase
GCS	Glasgow Coma Score
GI	gastrointestinal
GORD	gastro-oesophageal reflux disease
GP	general practitioner
GTN	glyceryl trinitrate
H^+	hydrogen ion
Hb	haemoglobin
Hb S(C)	sickle cell disease *and/or* haemoglobin
HBV	hepatitis B virus
HCC	hepatocellular carcinoma
HCO_3	bicarbonate
HCV	hepatitis C virus
HIV	human immunodeficiency virus
HLA	human leukocyte antigen
HOCM	hypertrophic obstructive cardiomyopathy
HONK	hyperosmolar non-ketotic
HRCT	high resolution CT
HRT	hormone replacement therapy
HSV	herpes simplex virus
HTLV	human T-cell lymphoma *or* leukaemia virus
HUS	haemolytic-uraemic syndrome
IBD	inflammatory bowel disease
ICD	International Classification of Diseases
IDL	intermediate density lipoprotein
IF	intrinsic factor
Ig	immunoglobulin
IGF-I	insulin-like growth factor-I
IHD	ischaemic heart disease
IM	intramuscular
INR	international normalised ratio
ITU	intensive care unit

IU	International Unit
IV	intravenous
ivou	intravenous drug user
IVP	intravenous pyelography
IVU	intravenous urography
K	potassium
kg	kilogram
kPa	kilopascal
l	litre
LDH	lactate dehydrogenase
LDL	low density lipoprotein
LFT	liver function test
LH	luteinising hormone
LHRH	luteinising hormone-releasing hormone
LMN	lower motor neurone
LMWH	low molecular weight heparin
MAOI	monoamine oxidase inhibitor
MC+S	microculture and sensitivity
mcg	microgram
MCH	mean cell *or* corpuscular haemoglobin
MCHC	mean cell haemoglobin count *or* concentration
MCQ	multiple choice question
MCV	mean cell *or* corpuscular volume
MDRTB	multi-drug resistant TB
MEN	multiple endocrine neoplasia
MEQ	modified essay question
mg	milligram
MI	myocardial infarction
mIBG	metaiodobenzylguanidine
MID	multi-infarct (vascular) dementia
MIE	meconium ileus equivalent
ml	millilitre
mmHg	millimetres of mercury
mmol/l	millimoles per litre
MODY	maturity-onset diabetes of the young
mOsmol/kg	milliosmoles per kilogram
MRI	magnetic resonance imaging
MSU	midstream urine
μg	microgram

μmol/l	micromoles per litre
Na	sodium
NaCl	sodium chloride
NaHCO$_3$	sodium bicarbonate
NGT	nasogastric tube
NICE	National Institute for Health and Clinical Excellence
nmol/l	nanomoles per litre
NSAID	non-steroidal anti-inflammatory drug
NSU	nonspecific urethritis
O$_2$	oxygen
OCP	oral contraceptive pill
OGD	oesophagogastroduodenoscopy
OSAHS	obstructive sleep apnoea/hypopnoea syndrome
OSCE	Objective Structured Clinical Examination
PA	posteroanterior
pa(CO$_2$)	partial pressure of carbon dioxide
pa(O$_2$)	partial pressure of oxygen
PAN	polyarteritis nodosa
PCOS	polycystic ovary syndrome
PCWP	pulmonary capillary wedge pressure
PE	pulmonary embolism
PEFR	peak expiratory flow rate
pg	picogram
po	*per os* (by mouth)
PPI	proton pump inhibitor
PR	*per rectum*
PRV	polycythaemia rubra vera
PTH	parathyroid hormone
PVD	peripheral *or* pulmonary vascular disease
RBG	random blood glucose
RSV	respiratory syncytial virus
SAQ	structured answer question
SDAT	senile dementia of the Alzheimer's type
SIADH	syndrome of inappropriate ADH
SLE	systemic lupus erythematosus
SNRI	serotonin–norepinephrine re-uptake inhibitor
STD	sexually transmitted disease
STEMI	ST elevation MI
SVT	supraventricular tachycardia

TB	tuberculosis
TENS	transcutaneous electrical nerve stimulation
TFT	thyroid function test
TG	triglyceride
TIA	transient ischaemic attack
TIBC	total iron-binding capacity
TIPSS	transjugular intrahepatic portal systemic shunt
tPA	tissue-type plasminogen activator
TPHA	*Treponema pallidum* haemagglutination assay
TRH	thyrotrophin-releasing hormone
TSH	thyroid-stimulating hormone
TTP	thrombotic thrombocytopenic purpura
TURP	transurethral resection of the prostate
U&E	urea & electrolytes
U1RNP	U1 ribonuclear protein
UMN	upper motor neurone
US(S)	ultrasound (scan)
UTI	urinary tract infection
UV	ultraviolet
V/Q	ventilation-perfusion
VATS	video-assisted thorascopic surgery
vCJD	variant Creutzfeldt–Jakob disease
VDRL	venereal disease research laboratory test
VER	visual evoked response
VF	ventricular fibrillation
VLDL	very low density lipoprotein
VT	ventricular tachycardia
WBC	white blood cell count
WCC	white cell count
WHO	World Health Organization

PART ONE

Structured Answer Questions

QUESTIONS

Infectious Diseases

Question 1

A 23-year-old medical student presents to the Emergency Department with a few hours' history of fever, rigors, vomiting, headache and severe myalgia affecting the lower limbs and trunk. She has just returned from elective studies in New Zealand, having spent the last week on a fresh water canoeing trip. On examination she has a temperature of 39.7°C but no signs of meningism.

(a) State the most likely diagnosis and the organism responsible **(3 marks)**

(b) List two possible treatments **(2 marks)**

(c) List five clinical features of the severe form of this illness **(5 marks)**

Question 2

A 45-year-old woman is referred to the rheumatology clinic with a year's history of intermittent joint stiffness affecting her right knee. On examination there is an effusion on the affected knee but no other abnormality. The patient recalls a slowly spreading, circular, red rash with central clearing, that appeared on her right leg after returning from a walking holiday in Denmark 18 months previously.

(a) What is: (i) the diagnosis, (ii) the causative organism, (iii) the vector and (iv) the name of the rash?

(4 marks)

(b) List four other manifestations of this disease   *(4 marks)*

(c) List two possible treatments   *(2 marks)*

Question 3

A 34-year-old man known to be HIV positive for ten years, and non-adherent to antiretroviral therapy, presents to the Emergency Department with a fortnight's history of increasing breathlessness associated with dry cough, malaise and fever. Chest X-ray shows bilateral perihilar interstitial shadowing.

(a) State the probable diagnosis and give a list of other possibilities   *(3 marks)*

(b) Outline the steps involved in diagnosis   *(4 marks)*

(c) Outline the treatment of the most probable diagnosis   *(3 marks)*

Question 4

A 43-year-old man with advanced HIV disease and a CD4 lymphocyte count of 20/mm³ is brought to the Emergency Department in a confused state. His partner tells you he has been complaining of headache and difficulty using his left hand for the past week. On examination he is pyrexial, incoherent, failing to obey commands and moving only his right side. Reflexes are normal on the right but brisk on the left with an upgoing plantar response.

(a) Which three components of examination, essential to a full neurological assessment of this patient, have been omitted from the description of findings? *(1 mark)*

(b) What is (i) the most likely diagnosis and (ii) its treatment? *(4 marks)*

(c) List five other conditions affecting the central nervous system that are characteristic of advanced HIV disease *(5 marks)*

Question 5

A 29-year-old Thai restaurateur presents to his GP with a three-month history of worsening jaundice and right upper quadrant pain. As an infant in Thailand he had been jaundiced, but had enjoyed good health until this present episode.

(a) What is the likely cause of his jaundice? *(1 mark)*

(b) List three modes of acquiring this disorder *(3 marks)*

(c) Briefly outline your investigations and therapeutic management *(6 marks)*

Question 6

A 13-year-old schoolgirl presents to the Emergency Department with a five-day history of an upper respiratory tract infection, now complicated by a severe headache, photophobia and neck stiffness. Her mother has also noticed a rapidly developing purpuric rash over her legs in the last few hours.

(a) State the diagnosis and list two possible causative organisms *(3 marks)*

(b) List six investigations you would perform *(3 marks)*

(c) Briefly outline your therapeutic management *(4 marks)*

Question 7

A 46-year-old woman returns from Bangladesh after a three-month visit to see her family. Whilst in Bangladesh she developed night sweats, a productive cough, with green sputum and occasional haemoptysis. In the last two weeks she has also developed diarrhoea and has lost several kg in weight.

(a) What is the likely organism causing her symptoms? *(1 mark)*

(b) List five investigations that you would perform in this case to confirm the diagnosis *(5 marks)*

(c) List the drugs that may be used in this case, with a side-effect of each *(4 marks)*

Question 8

A 36-year-old man presents to his GP three days after returning from a business trip to Nigeria, with a five-day history of fever, malaise and rigors. He denies any other systemic upset and has not taken any antimalarial prophylaxis.

(a) List three species of malaria and three drugs used in the treatment *(3 marks)*

(b) List three investigations that you would perform *(3 marks)*

(c) Outline the advice that you would have given this man if he had come to see you prior to his trip *(4 marks)*

Question 9

A 17-year-old schoolgirl presents to her GP with a two-week history of worsening pharyngitis associated with flu-like symptoms and swelling of the lymph nodes in her neck. On examination she has a petechial rash over her soft palate, tender cervical lymphadenopathy and splenomegaly, with the spleen palpable 2 cm below the left costal margin.

(a) State the most likely infectious cause of her symptoms and give two alternative diagnoses *(3 marks)*

(b) List five investigations you would perform *(5 marks)*

(c) Outline your management *(2 marks)*

Question 10

A 24-year-old businessman returns from Bangkok with a one-week history of a painful urethral discharge and a painless ulcerative lesion on the glans of his penis.

(a) (i)   What is the term used to describe the lesion on his penis? *(1 mark)*

        (ii)   List two organisms that may be responsible for his symptoms *(2 marks)*

(b) Give three other examples of infectious diseases that may be acquired in a similar manner *(3 marks)*

(c) Outline your investigations and therapeutic management *(4 marks)*

Question 11

A 21-year-old man presents to the Emergency Department with an eight-hour history of diarrhoea and abdominal cramps, after eating some poorly thawed chicken at a barbecue.

(a) (i)   What is the condition from which he is suffering? *(1 mark)*

        (ii)   List three organisms that could be responsible *(3 marks)*

(b) Give two other risk factors for contracting such an illness *(2 marks)*

(c) Briefly outline your investigations and therapeutic management *(4 marks)*

Question 12

A 59-year-old man is recovering five days after an elective right total hip replacement. He has an indwelling urinary catheter in situ and an intravenous cannula in each forearm. During the last 24 hours he has become increasingly unwell, with a swinging pyrexia. He is now clammy and pale, with a pulse of 110 beats per minute and a blood pressure of 80/60 mmHg.

(a) (i) What is the term used to describe his condition?
(1 mark)
(ii) List three possible causes in this man's case
(3 marks)

(b) List six essential investigations that you would perform
(3 marks)

(c) Briefly outline your management
(3 marks)

Question 13

A 21-year-old female nurse returns from working in India with a two-month history of diarrhoea, now associated with episodic rigors and right upper quadrant pain. She also complains of an irritating pain in her right shoulder. Stool culture and microscopy reveal cysts.

(a) What is the diagnosis and the causative organism?
(2 marks)

(b) What is the cause of her right upper quadrant pain? How is it related to her shoulder pain?
(2 marks)

(c) (i) List three investigations that you would perform in this case
(3 marks)
(ii) Outline the therapeutic options
(3 marks)

Question 14

A 27-year-old man returns after a two-year period working in Thailand, with a three-month history of intermittent abdominal pain, diarrhoea and a dry cough associated with wheezing. During this period he has lost 5 kg in weight. A full blood count organised by his GP shows a normal white cell count but with a 'gross eosinophilia'.

(a) (i) What is the likely group of organisms responsible for his eosinophilia? *(1 mark)*

      (ii) List two other causes of an eosinophilia *(2 marks)*

(b) What is the cause of his respiratory symptoms?

(2 marks)

(c) Briefly outline your investigations and therapeutic management *(5 marks)*

Question 15

A 19-year-old student returns from a caving holiday in the southern states of America with a two-week history of fever, a non-productive cough and arthralgia. His GP sends him to the chest clinic where a diagnosis of histoplasmosis is made.

(a) (i) What type of organism is *Histoplasma*? *(1 mark)*

      (ii) List two more common conditions that are caused by this group of organisms *(2 marks)*

(b) List three investigations that you would perform *(3 marks)*

(c) List four drugs used in the treatment of such infections, with a side-effect of each *(4 marks)*

2

Metabolic Diseases

Question 1

A 28-year-old Somalian woman presents to her GP with a two-year history of bone pains and proximal muscle weakness. She has taken carbamazepine for epilepsy for the past five years and lives with her three small children in a women's refuge. On examination there is mild kyphosis but no other abnormality.

(a) State the diagnosis *(1 mark)*

(b) List the factors contributing to the development of this condition *(5 marks)*

(c) Outline your management *(4 marks)*

Question 2

A 16-year-old schoolboy presents to the medical outpatient department with a three-month history of neurological symptoms, including tremor, and choreiform movements, associated with behavioural problems at school. On examination he has several stigmata of chronic liver disease, and greyish rings are noted around the cornea. A clinical diagnosis of Wilson's disease is made.

(a) What is the name given to the grey corneal rings and which trace element is associated with this disorder? *(2 marks)*

(b) List three investigations that would confirm the clinical diagnosis *(3 marks)*

(c) Outline your therapeutic management *(5 marks)*

Question 3

A 36-year-old man presents to his GP with a three-month history of polyuria and polydipsia, associated with painful swelling of both knees. On examination he has a suntanned appearance (despite not having been in the sun for several months), and has several signs of chronic liver disease, with 5 cm hepatomegaly below the right costal margin. He also has arthritis of both knees.

(a) State the diagnosis and the causative factor *(3 marks)*

(b) List five investigations that you would perform *(4 marks)*

(c) What is the cause of:
(i) the polyuria and polydipsia?
(ii) his suntanned appearance?
(iii) the arthritis? *(3 marks)*

Question 4

A 27-year-old man is found to have a cholesterol of 11.0 mmol/l with normal triglycerides, at a routine insurance medical examination. On direct questioning he says that his father and uncle, both non-smokers, died in their early 40s of ischaemic heart disease.

(a) Which inherited disorder does this man have and what is its mode of inheritance?   *(2 marks)*

(b) List two clinical signs you would look for in association with this cholesterol level, and two bedside tests that you would perform   *(4 marks)*

(c) Briefly outline your management   *(4 marks)*

Question 5

A two-year-old boy with known glucose-6-phosphatase deficiency presents in the Paediatric Outpatient Department with increasing lethargy and general ill health. On examination he is of short stature and obese; he has hepatomegaly and palpable kidneys.

(a) Of which group of disorders is this disease an example?   *(2 marks)*

(b) What is its mode of inheritance? Give three other examples   *(4 marks)*

(c) If this patient was presenting for the first time, how would you attempt to confirm the diagnosis (definitive tests are not required)   *(4 marks)*

Question 6

A 20-year-old woman presents to the Emergency Department with a six-hour history of acute abdominal pain. She denies any gastrointestinal or urogenital symptoms, but says she has had two less severe, similar episodes in the last few months since starting the oral contraceptive pill. The medical registrar makes a clinical diagnosis of acute porphyria.

(a) Give two further symptoms that may be presenting features *(2 marks)*

(b) List three other precipitating factors *(3 marks)*

(c) Outline your therapeutic management *(5 marks)*

Question 7

A 3-year-old boy is brought to the Paediatric Outpatient Department by his parents, who are both Ashkenazi Jews. The boy has been unwell for several months complaining of left upper quadrant abdominal pain. On examination he is clinically anaemic, has a greyish pigmentation and has multiple bruises over his back and forearms. He is also noted to have hepatomegaly and massive splenomegaly. A clinical diagnosis of Gaucher's disease is made.

(a) List two other disorders that are common amongst Ashkenazi Jews *(2 marks)*

(b) (i) To which group of disorders does Gaucher's disease belong and what is its mode of inheritance? *(2 marks)*
 (ii) List three investigations that are indicated from the history *(3 marks)*

(c) Outline your advice to the parents with regard to treatment and prognosis *(3 marks)*

Question 8

A 21-year-old man with known homocystinuria presents to the Emergency Department with a 36-hour history of increasing pain and swelling in the left calf, now associated with shortness of breath and an episode of haemoptysis. On examination he has Marfanoid features with pectus carinatum.

(a) What is the mode of inheritance of this disorder?

(1 mark)

(b) List three Marfanoid features and explain the term pectus carinatum

(4 marks)

(c) What is the presenting complication in this case? Briefly outline your therapeutic management

(5 marks)

Question 9

A previously healthy 17-year-old girl was admitted to the Emergency Department following an overdose of aspirin. On examination she was semi-conscious, hypotensive and oliguric.

(a) List the metabolic effects of salicylate toxicity

(3 marks)

(b) How would you correct the metabolic deficit?

(4 marks)

(c) List three other drugs with similar toxic effects

(3 marks)

Question 10

A 29-year-old female athlete collapsed during the London Marathon. She was taken to the Emergency Department where she was found to be conscious but hyperventilating and hypotensive.

(a) State the main physiological events that had overcome the patient and their underlying mechanisms *(4 marks)*

(b) List the immediate resuscitatory measures required *(2 marks)*

(c) How would you assess and correct the underlying metabolic disorder? *(4 marks)*

3

Neurology

Question 1

A 74-year-old man is sent to the Emergency Department by his GP with a six to seven-hour history of weakness affecting his left upper and lower limbs, and the left side of his face. He also complains of slurring of his speech.

(a) What is the diagnosis and which blood vessel is most likely to be involved? *(2 marks)*

(b) List the clinical features you would use to differentiate between an upper and a lower motor neurone weakness *(2 marks)*

(c) List the essential investigations you would perform *(3 marks)*
and outline your further management *(3 marks)*

Question 2

A 19-year-old secretary presents to the Emergency Department with a six-hour history of a severe headache. The headache came on suddenly whilst she was at work. She says she feels as though 'someone has hit me over the back of the head with a baseball bat'. She has been nauseated with mild neck stiffness, but denies fever or photophobia.

(a) What is the likely cause of her headache?   *(1 mark)*

(b) Give three other causes of a severe headache in this case   *(3 marks)*

(c) Briefly outline your investigations and therapeutic management   *(6 marks)*

Question 3

A 59-year-old smoker presents to his GP with a four-month history of a cough, episodic haemoptysis, and a 10 kg weight loss. On examination he has a partial ptosis of the right eye associated with enophthalmos and a constricted pupil. Respiratory examination reveals coarse crackles and bronchial breathing in the right upper zone.

(a) What is the eponymous syndrome associated with this man's eye signs, and what is the neurological lesion involved?   *(2 marks)*

(b) (i)   What is the probable cause of the syndrome
          in this case?   *(1 mark)*
    (ii) List three other causes   *(3 marks)*

(c) Another patient presents with a full ptosis and fixed dilated pupil of the right eye. The eye is facing down and out. Explain neurologically the appearances of the eye and list two causes   *(4 marks)*

Question 4

A 47-year-old woman presents to her GP with a two-day history of a weakness affecting the left side of her face. She has no other neurological deficit and is otherwise well.

(a) (i)   Which cranial nerve has been affected?   *(1 mark)*

(ii) How would you differentiate between an upper and a lower motor neurone lesion?   *(2 marks)*

(b) List four causes of this cranial nerve palsy   *(4 marks)*

(c) It is suspected this is an idiopathic lower motor neurone lesion. What is the eponymous name of this lesion? Briefly outline your management   *(3 marks)*

Question 5

A 36-year-old man with known poorly controlled insulin-dependent diabetes mellitus presents in the diabetic clinic with a three-month history of worsening numbness and paraesthesiae in his hands and feet, associated with a large ulcer on the sole of his left heel.

(a) (i)   What is the probable cause of his symptoms?
   (1 mark)

(ii) List two other causes   *(2 marks)*

(b) List the modalities of sensation that you would test and the spinal tracts in which they are carried   *(3 marks)*

(c) List four other neurological complications of diabetes mellitus   *(4 marks)*

Question 6

A 26-year-old woman presents to her GP with a two-month history of early morning headaches. The headaches are constant, but far worse in the mornings and when she laughs or coughs. Initially they were relieved by aspirin but now nothing seems to make the headache better. More recently she has been nauseated and has had some blurring of her vision.

(a) List three possible causes of her headache *(3 marks)*

(b) Give three essential investigations you would perform in this case *(3 marks)*

(c) Outline the therapeutic options *(4 marks)*

Question 7

A 20-year-old female student presents in the neurology outpatient department with a three-month history of 'funny turns' lasting two to three minutes. Each is preceded by an 'odd sensation', and is followed by a feeling of 'vacancy'. She has no recollection of these events, but has been told about them by her friends, who say she becomes vacant and unresponsive, with grinding of her teeth and contortion of her face.

(a) What is the likely cause of her 'turns'? *(1 mark)*

(b) List five investigations that you would perform *(5 marks)*

(c) List four therapeutic agents that may be used in this case, giving a side-effect of each *(4 marks)*

Question 8

A 57-year-old man is seen in the Neurology Outpatient Department with a four-month history of wasting of his upper and lower limbs, associated with progressive worsening of his mobility. More recently he has also had 'difficulty' with his speech and 'choking' whilst eating and drinking.

(a) What is the underlying diagnosis, and the reason for his 'difficulty' with speech and 'choking' when eating?

(3 marks)

(b) List three investigations relevant to this case *(3 marks)*

(c) List the management strategies you would use

(4 marks)

Question 9

A 29-year-old woman presents to her GP with a four-month history of shoulder and hip weakness, particularly with exercise. She has also noticed blurring of her vision and difficulty with chewing, particularly towards the end of a long meal. The most striking feature on examination is marked bilateral ptosis, with weakness of the extra-ocular muscles.

(a) State the diagnosis and its pathogenesis *(3 marks)*

(b) List two investigations that you would perform *(2 marks)*

(c) List the therapeutic options that you would employ

(5 marks)

Question 10

A 62-year-old man presents to the Medical Outpatients Department with a one-year history of progressive difficulty in walking and falls. He has developed a marked tremor of both hands and has noticed that his writing is becoming increasingly 'shaky and small'.

(a) What is the diagnosis and the neurotransmitter involved in this condition?   *(2 marks)*

(b) List two other conditions that may present in a similar manner   *(2 marks)*

(c) List three drugs that may be used in this case and a recognised side-effect of each   *(6 marks)*

Question 11

A three-year-old boy presents in the paediatric clinic with repeated falls, poor walking and an inability to climb on to furniture or up the stairs. A clinical diagnosis of Duchenne's muscular dystrophy is made.

(a) (i)   How is this disorder classically inherited?
          (1 mark)

(ii) List two other examples of this type of inheritance   *(2 marks)*

(b) List three investigations to confirm the clinical diagnosis in this patient   *(3 marks)*

(c) List four other causes of proximal muscle weakness
          (4 marks)

Question 12

A 26-year-old man is sent to the Neurology Outpatient Department by his GP with an eight-week history of numbness and paraesthesiae in his hands and feet, associated with an episode of blurred vision and pain in the left eye which resolved spontaneously.

(a) What is the underlying diagnosis, and what is the pathological basis of the disorder? *(2 marks)*

(b) List three investigations that you would perform and the expected abnormalities *(3 marks)*

(c) Briefly outline your management once the diagnosis is confirmed *(5 marks)*

Question 13

A 62-year-old woman presents to the Emergency Department with a two-week history of increasing weakness and numbness in her lower limbs, associated with difficulty in passing urine and constipation. She had a Dukes' C carcinoma of the colon treated 18 months previously. On examination she has a spastic paraparesis and a sensory loss at level T10.

(a) (i) What is the likely cause of the spastic paraparesis in this case? *(1 mark)*
    (ii) List two other causes *(2 marks)*

(b) Define the surface anatomy of a T10 sensory level and list three essential investigations that you would perform to confirm the lesion and its level *(4 marks)*

(c) Outline your management strategy *(3 marks)*

Question 14

A 27-year-old man presents to the Emergency Department with a ten-day history of an upper respiratory tract infection, now associated with increasing weakness and numbness in the lower limbs. On examination he has lower motor neurone signs in his lower limbs associated with sensory loss to the level of the upper thighs.

(a) (i) What is the cause of this man's sensorimotor
neuropathy? *(1 mark)*
(ii) List two other causes *(2 marks)*

(b) List the lower motor neurone signs that you
would elicit *(3 marks)*

(c) Outline your therapeutic management *(4 marks)*

Question 15

A 45-year-old man is brought to the Neurology Outpatient Department by his wife, with an eight-month history of increasing forgetfulness, inappropriately aggressive behaviour and a generalised change in his personality. More recently he has had 'writhing' and 'lunging' movements of the arms and legs. His wife thinks his father also had a similar problem. A clinical diagnosis of Huntington's chorea is made.

(a) How is this disorder inherited and what are the chances
of this man's offspring being affected? *(2 marks)*

(b) Define what is meant by chorea and give two other
causes *(4 marks)*

(c) Briefly outline your management *(4 marks)*

Question 16

A 49-year-old man, who is a known chronic alcohol abuser, presents to the Emergency Department with a two-day history of worsening tremor and decreased mobility. He has been on phenytoin for two years after sustaining a head injury whilst inebriated. On examination he has several stigmata of chronic liver disease and gross cerebellar signs. He is not encephalopathic.

(a) List four cerebellar signs you may expect to elicit

(2 marks)

(b) Give two causes of the cerebellar syndrome in this patient

(2 marks)

(c) List three investigations that you would perform and three drugs you would prescribe in this man's further management

(6 marks)

4

Endocrinology

Question 1

A 19-year-old man with poorly controlled type I diabetes mellitus is brought to the Emergency Department in a semi-comatose state.

(a) List (i) two diabetic emergencies to consider in reaching a diagnosis and (ii) two other metabolic emergencies resulting from diabetes mellitus or its treatment   *(2 marks)*

(b) His capillary blood glucose is 25.7 mmol/l. List four other urgent investigations, explaining each choice
                                                                (2 marks)

(c) Outline your acute management   *(6 marks)*

Question 2

A 27-year-old body builder is found to be oligozoospermic during investigations for infertility, having already had a child with a previous partner. He denies erectile dysfunction and describes having undergone normal puberty. On examination he has very prominent musculature and atrophic testes but secondary sexual characteristics are otherwise normal.

(a) State the likely cause of the oligozoospermia   *(1 mark)*

(b) List five other causes of male infertility   *(5 marks)*

(c) Outline your approach to making the diagnosis
                                             (4 marks)

Question 3

A 22-year-old woman presents to her GP with long-standing acne and facial hirsutism that she plucks daily. Her periods are irregular. On examination she is overweight with mild axillary and cervical acanthosis nigricans. There is pigmented hair in the beard area and escutcheon but she is not virilised.

(a) State her diagnosis and a differential   *(2 marks)*

(b) List the relevant investigations   *(4 marks)*

(c) Outline your management   *(4 marks)*

Question 4

A 58-year-old woman gives a year's history of cold intolerance, lethargy, constipation, reduced appetite and weight gain. Serum free thyroxine and free triiodothyronine levels are low and serum thyroid stimulating hormone is grossly elevated.

(a) (i) State the clinical diagnosis (*1 mark*)
    (ii) List four causes of this condition (*2 marks*)

(b) Discuss the therapeutic management of this patient
(*3 marks*)

(c) Before treatment could commence, the patient was found unconscious at home. Discuss your management
(*4 marks*)

Question 5

A 31-year-old woman is referred to the Medical Clinic with a history of heat intolerance, fatigue, palpitations and weight loss despite a voracious appetite. On examination she has a fine tremor and proptosis.

(a) State the probable clinical diagnosis and its pathogenesis (*3 marks*)

(b) List the other clinical findings that would confirm your diagnosis (*3 marks*)

(c) List the treatment modalities available and their complications (*4 marks*)

Question 6

A 36-year-old woman is referred to the Endocrinology Clinic with a history of galactorrhoea and secondary amenorrhoea. She is not taking any medication. Visual fields are normal. Her serum prolactin level is elevated.

(a) (i) State the likely pathological cause   *(1 mark)*
(ii) State a differential diagnosis   *(1 mark)*

(b) List four drugs that may elevate plasma prolactin
        (4 marks)

(c) Outline your investigation and treatment of the likely pathological cause   *(4 marks)*

Question 7

A 45-year-old woman is referred to the Endocrine Clinic with a history of joint pains, coarsening of her facial features and recent-onset type II diabetes mellitus. Over the last two years her shoe size has increased and she has had to have her wedding ring enlarged.

(a) (i) State the clinical diagnosis and probable pathological cause   *(2 marks)*
(ii) State the cardinal diagnostic test and the expected result   *(2 marks)*

(b) List six other clinical features that characterise this disease   *(3 marks)*

(c) List the methods of treating this condition   *(3 marks)*

Question 8

A 35-year-old woman with proximal myopathy, easy bruising, hypertension and central obesity is diagnosed as having Cushing's syndrome.

(a) State (i) the pathological basis of Cushing's syndrome and (ii) four potential causes *(3 marks)*

(b) List six other clinical features of Cushing's syndrome *(3 marks)*

(c) List (i) two biochemical tests used to confirm the presence of Cushing's syndrome and (ii) two biochemical tests used to establish the underlying cause *(4 marks)*

Question 9

A 58-year-old woman with a six-month history of weight loss, malaise, weakness and skin hyperpigmentation is found to be suffering from primary adrenal insufficiency.

(a) State (i) the eponymous term for primary adrenal insufficiency and (ii) four causes of this condition *(3 marks)*

(b) List six more clinical features associated with this condition *(3 marks)*

(c) List (i) two abnormalities on serum urea and electrolyte testing that are characteristic of primary adrenal insufficiency and (ii) two biochemical tests that provide confirmation of the clinical diagnosis *(4 marks)*

CHAPTER 4 – QUESTIONS

Question 10

*A 60-year-old man presents with severe
hypertension associated with muscle weakness.
A diagnosis of primary hyperaldosteronism is made.*

(a) State the pathophysiology of this disease   *(4 marks)*

(b) State three diagnostic biochemical findings   *(3 marks)*

(c) State the principles of treatment   *(3 marks)*

Question 11

*A 29-year-old woman complains to her GP of
increased thirst and urine production. Her renal
function, electrolytes and plasma glucose are
normal. In a subsequent water deprivation test, she
rapidly becomes dehydrated while continuing to
pass large quantities of dilute urine, but responds
appropriately to desmopressin (DDAVP).*

(a) What is an appropriate response to desmopressin?
(3 marks)

(b) State (i) her diagnosis and (ii) list the options for
treatment   *(4 marks)*

(c) List three possible underlying causes of this diagnosis
(3 marks)

Question 12

A 52-year-old woman complains to her GP of polyuria, fatigue and constipation and is found to be hypercalcaemic with a corrected serum calcium of 3.0 mmol/l. Her renal function and serum vitamin D level are normal but the serum parathyroid hormone and urinary calcium are both elevated. She is referred to the endocrine clinic.

(a) State (i) what is meant by a 'corrected' serum calcium and (ii) the patient's likely diagnosis   *(2 marks)*

(b) List six other causes of hypercalcaemia   *(3 marks)*

(c) Whilst waiting for her endocrine appointment, a locum GP prescribes her bendrofluazide for hypertension. A week later she is admitted as an emergency with dehydration, confusion and a serum calcium of 4.2 mmol/l. Outline your management   *(5 marks)*

Question 13

A 49-year-old man complains of paroxysmal attacks of headache, palpitations, vomiting, breathlessness and weakness, and says he felt he was 'going to die' during the episodes. Clinically he is pale and hypertensive.

(a) List four differential diagnoses that would fit the above findings   *(2 marks)*

(b) His plasma and urinary adrenaline levels are grossly elevated. State (i) the diagnosis and (ii) your strategy for localising the lesion   *(5 marks)*

(c) Outline your treatment   *(3 marks)*

Question 14

A 21-year-old woman, with a history of obesity and polycystic ovary syndrome, presents to her GP with a 5-week history of polyuria, polydipsia and 10 kg weight loss. Her capillary blood glucose is above the reference range of the surgery's meter.

(a) State three possible diagnoses   *(3 marks)*

(b) How would you confirm the diagnosis?   *(3 marks)*

(c) Outline your approach to treatment   *(4 marks)*

Question 15

A 54-year-old man presents to his GP complaining of a three-month history of thirst, blurred vision and tiredness. On examination he is obese and has retinopathy in a pattern suggestive of diabetes mellitus. Random plasma glucose is 16.1 mmol/l.

(a) Outline the classification of diabetic retinopathy and give a principal feature of each grade   *(3 marks)*

(b) Give six other common presenting symptoms of diabetes mellitus   *(3 marks)*

(c) List four classes of antidiabetic medication and give an example of each   *(4 marks)*

Respiratory Medicine

Question 1

A 28-year-old alcoholic of no fixed abode presents to the Emergency Department with a three-day history of fever, rigors, shortness of breath, pleuritic right-sided chest pain and expectoration of blood-stained, brown sputum. On examination he is pyrexial and has chest signs compatible with a right-sided pleural effusion.

(a) List the characteristic signs of a pleural effusion

(3 marks)

(b) State (i) the two most likely types of effusion and (ii) the underlying diagnosis *(3 marks)*

(c) Outline your management *(4 marks)*

Question 2

A 55-year-old obese man undergoes open reduction and internal fixation of a lower limb fracture sustained after falling asleep at the wheel of his bus. Extubation is difficult and it is subsequently noted that, whilst sleeping, he has a disrupted breathing pattern with frequent prolonged pauses.

(a) State (i) his diagnosis, and (ii) three characteristic symptoms *(4 marks)*

(b) List the consequences of this condition *(3 marks)*

(c) Outline your management *(3 marks)*

Question 3

A 25-year-old man presents to the Emergency Department with left-sided pleuritic chest pain and mild dyspnoea that began suddenly after sneezing. There are no other symptoms. He is a smoker and has a history of asthma for which he uses salbutamol and beclomethasone inhalers. On examination his temperature, pulse and blood pressure are normal. Breath sounds are vesicular but reduced on the left side.

(a) State the probable diagnosis *(1 mark)*

(b) While waiting in the department, the patient's breathing suddenly and rapidly deteriorates. State (i) the complication that is likely to have occurred and (ii) six clinical signs that support the diagnosis *(4 marks)*

(c) Outline your management *(5 marks)*

Question 4

A 67-year-old retired electrician is referred to outpatients with an 8-week history of gradually increasing shortness of breath. Over the preceding 6 months he has been aware of a continuous dull ache in the left shoulder. He has lost two stones in weight over the same period. There is no past medical history, he is not on any medication, and he has not smoked since the birth of his first child 40 years ago. A chest radiograph shows a large left pleural effusion.

(a) Mesothelioma is suspected. List six other causes of unilateral pleural effusion   *(3 marks)*

(b) List the tests that should be undertaken on a diagnostic aspirate of the pleural effusion, and indicate the expected results   *(4 marks)*

(c) A firm diagnosis is not reached after diagnostic aspiration. List three other investigations which may be helpful   *(3 marks)*

Question 5

A 17-year-old male student with known asthma attends the Emergency Department with a three-day history of a cough productive of yellow sputum, worsening shortness of breath and wheeze.

(a) Give two reasons why a chest X-ray must be performed
(*2 marks*)

(b) List three other investigations that you would perform
(*3 marks*)

(c) (i) List the criteria that you would use to assess the severity of this asthma exacerbation (*2 marks*)
(ii) Briefly outline your initial therapeutic management (*3 marks*)

Question 6

A 26-year-old woman presents to her GP with a three-day history of a dry cough and exertional dyspnoea. A chest X-ray reveals 'patchy consolidation' in the right upper lobe for which she is started on amoxicillin. Over the next 48 hours she continues to deteriorate and is subsequently admitted to hospital.

(a) What is the descriptive term given to this woman's condition? (*1 mark*)

(b) List four causative organisms that may be implicated
(*4 marks*)

(c) State an expected abnormality in each of the following investigations: (i) FBC, (ii) U&Es, (iii) LFTs, (iv) ABGs and (v) immune markers (*5 marks*)

Question 7

A 63-year-old man who is a lifelong smoker attends the chest clinic with a two- to three-year history of worsening exertional dyspnoea, associated with a productive cough. He is prone to chest infections during the winter months.

(a) Outline the important points you would need to elucidate in the history *(5 marks)*

(b) List three non-haematological investigations you would do in this case *(3 marks)*

(c) List four drugs that may be employed in this case *(2 marks)*

Question 8

A 61-year-old man presents to his GP with a four-month history of a cough associated with episodic fresh haemoptysis. During this period he has lost 5 kg in weight despite a reasonable appetite. He is a lifelong smoker.

(a) What is the most likely diagnosis? *(1 mark)*

(b) List three investigations to confirm the diagnosis *(3 marks)*

(c) Describe the various treatment options *(6 marks)*

Question 9

A 28-year-old woman presents to the Emergency Department with a six-hour history of sudden onset of severe, right-sided pleuritic chest pain, associated with shortness of breath and an episode of haemoptysis.

(a) What is the most likely diagnosis? *(1 mark)*

(b) List six risk factors for this disease *(3 marks)*

(c) (i) Outline the investigations that you would perform *(3 marks)*
(ii) Briefly outline the therapeutic management *(3 marks)*

Question 10

A 30-year-old Black-Caribbean woman presents to her GP with a six-month history of exertional dyspnoea, and a painful red lesion on her shin. She also complains of dry itchy eyes. A clinical diagnosis of sarcoidosis is made.

(a) What is the painful red lesion on her shin, and what is the term used to describe her eye condition? *(2 marks)*

(b) List three other extra-pulmonary manifestations of sarcoidosis *(3 marks)*

(c) List the essential investigations to confirm the diagnosis *(5 marks)*

Question 11

A 16-year-old schoolboy with a known chronic chest condition presents to his GP with a three-month history of worsening malaise, lethargy and loose, offensive, porridge-like stools. On examination he is pale and cachectic, with marked clubbing of his fingernails. Respiratory examination reveals an expiratory wheeze associated with coarse bibasal crackles and production of copious amounts of green sputum. His BM is 17–28 mmol/l.

(a) What is the chronic underlying disorder? *(1 mark)*

(b) Which three complications have developed? *(3 marks)*

(c) List the long-term management strategies that you would employ in the management *(6 marks)*

Question 12

A 55-year-old man presents to the chest clinic with a 12-month history of worsening exertional dyspnoea associated with an irritating dry cough. On examination he has clubbing of the fingernails and fine inspiratory crepitations are heard in the lower zones of both lung fields.

(a) What is the diagnosis? *(1 mark)*

(b) List three disorders that may present or are associated with this diagnosis *(3 marks)*

(c) List three investigations to confirm the diagnosis and the expected abnormality with each *(6 marks)*

Question 13

A 66-year-old retired boiler lagger presents to his GP with a three-month history of worsening shortness of breath and, more recently, a cough with episodic haemoptysis. He is a lifelong smoker.

(a) To which group of pulmonary disorders does this man's underlying condition belong? Give two other examples
(3 marks)

(b) What is the most likely cause of his shortness of breath and the haemoptysis? *(2 marks)*

(c) List the radiological features that may be seen on this man's chest X-ray *(5 marks)*

Question 14

A 32-year-old farm labourer presents to his GP with a six-month history of episodic shortness of breath associated with a flu-like illness. His symptoms are particularly prevalent when he is working with hay and straw.

(a) What is the condition from which he is suffering and to which group of pulmonary disorders does it belong?
(2 marks)

(b) List four agents or sources that have been implicated in the causation of these disorders *(4 marks)*

(c) Briefly outline your advice to this man if he decides to continue farming *(4 marks)*

Question 15

A 21-year-old female student is hit by a car whilst cycling home from college. She sustains multiple fractures, which are surgically reduced. During the post-operative 48 hours, her respiratory function worsens insidiously, and after review by the medical registrar she is electively intubated and ventilated.

(a) What is the term used to describe her respiratory problem? *(1 mark)*

(b) Give two diagnostic criteria *(2 marks)*

(c) (i) List six essential investigations that you would perform *(3 marks)*

(ii) Briefly outline your management prior to her being ventilated *(4 marks)*

6

Cardiology

Question 1

A 59-year-old man presents to the Emergency Department with a week's history of worsening of his usual angina pain. It is now occurring at rest in frequent episodes, each about 15 minutes long. A 12-lead ECG during pain shows ST depression in leads V2 to V6 and these changes resolve as the pain fades. Serum troponin I is negative on admission and again 12 hours later.

(a) State the diagnosis   *(2 marks)*

(b) List the treatments to be administered in the
Emergency Department   *(4 marks)*

(c) State the origin of troponin I and the relevance of the
results in this case   *(4 marks)*

Question 2

A 79-year-old, previously healthy woman presents to the Emergency Department with an acute inferior myocardial infarction. Whilst she is receiving thrombolytic therapy, her pulse slows down dramatically. A 12-lead ECG shows regular P-waves at 80 beats per minute and regular, narrow QRS complexes proceeding independently at 50 beats per minute.

(a) State the diagnosis   *(2 marks)*

(b) List four drugs, from at least two classes, that are contraindicated in this situation   *(4 marks)*

(c) The patient is not haemodynamically compromised. List four treatment options   *(4 marks)*

Question 3

A 25-year-old man presents to the Emergency Department with a short history of sharp, continuous, central chest pain that is worsened by deep inspiration and relieved by sitting upright. He has been troubled by intermittent fever and lethargy for the last few days but has no past medical history. On examination, a rub is heard during ventricular systole.

(a) State the diagnosis and three possible causative agents   *(4 marks)*

(b) Describe the characteristic ECG changes   *(3 marks)*

(c) List six non-infectious causes of a similar syndrome   *(3 marks)*

Question 4

A 41-year-old woman with a history of hypertension in pregnancy presents to the Emergency Department on the morning of New Year's Day with palpitations and dyspnoea which were present on waking. On examination she has a regular pulse of 150 beats per minute.

(a) List four possible electrocardiographic diagnoses

(4 marks)

(b) Give six possible underlying causes *(3 marks)*

(c) Outline your treatment of the most likely electrocardiographic diagnosis *(3 marks)*

Question 5

A 47-year-old man presents to the Emergency Department with a four-hour history of severe central chest pain radiating to his neck and arms. He is sweaty, nauseated and has felt dizzy and faint.

(a) (i) What is the most likely diagnosis? *(1 mark)*
    (ii) List six major risk factors *(2 marks)*

(b) List six drugs that have been proven to improve prognosis in this condition *(3 marks)*

(c) Briefly outline your management *(4 marks)*

Question 6

Six weeks after an acute anterior myocardial infarction, a 47-year-old man is seen in the medical outpatients department. Since discharge he has remained asymptomatic. Investigations whilst he was an inpatient show: glucose 15.4 mmol/l, cholesterol 7.6 mmol/l, normal triglycerides, echocardiogram 'moderately impaired left ventricular function'.

(a) List four drugs that you would ensure this man was taking *(4 marks)*

(b) Which other department in the hospital must he attend? *(1 mark)*

(c) Briefly outline your further management *(5 marks)*

Question 7

A 64-year-old retired headmistress presents to her GP with a three-month history of exertional dyspnoea, swelling of her ankles and orthopnoea even with three pillows at night. In the past she has had two myocardial infarctions, and remains on treatment for long-standing hypertension.

(a) Name two medications she may be taking which could be exacerbating her symptoms *(2 marks)*

(b) List the radiological features that may be evident on a CXR *(4 marks)*

(c) Briefly outline your management for this woman *(4 marks)*

Question 8

A 71-year-old retired policeman attends the medical outpatient department with a three-month history of episodic fast, irregular palpitations, associated with shortness of breath. On one occasion his left upper and lower limbs became weak, but this resolved spontaneously. He smokes ten cigarettes per day and drinks a half bottle of whisky every two days.

(a) (i) What is the likely tachyarrhythmia causing his symptoms?   *(1 mark)*

(ii) List two conditions that may be responsible for his arrhythmia, and his risk factors for developing them   *(2 marks)*

(b) What is the term used to describe the limb weakness?
(2 marks)

(c) Outline your management in this case   *(5 marks)*

Question 9

A 48-year-old factory manager presents to the Emergency Department with a three-week history of exertional dyspnoea, malaise and fever. During the 48 hours prior to presentation he has been in bed with a flu-like illness and a dry cough. His wife comments that his ankles have swelled markedly during this period. On examination he has a harsh pansystolic murmur, principally in the mitral area.

(a) (i) What is the underlying diagnosis?   *(1 mark)*

(ii) List three eponymous signs associated with the diagnosis, explaining what they are   *(3 marks)*

(b) Give two essential investigations that you would perform   *(2 marks)*

(c) List the complications that may occur   *(4 marks)*

Question 10

A 36-year-old keen amateur sportsman presents to the Cardiology Clinic with a six-month history of exertional dyspnoea, and chest pains, associated with one episode of collapse whilst out jogging. Of note his father had 'dropped dead' whilst playing football.

(a) What is the underlying cardiac condition and how is it inherited?   *(2 marks)*

(b) List three other causes of cardiomyopathy   *(3 marks)*

(c) Briefly outline your investigations and management
                                                      (5 marks)

Question 11

A 16-year-old schoolgirl presents to the Outpatient Department with worsening exertional dyspnoea. On examination she has marked clubbing of her fingernails and is cyanosed at rest. Cardiovascular examination reveals a parasternal heave and an ejection systolic murmur, heard predominantly in the pulmonary area.

(a) Give three causes of cyanotic heart disease   *(3 marks)*

(b) What are the four components of Fallot's tetralogy?
                                                      (4 marks)

(c) Briefly outline the treatment options   *(3 marks)*

Question 12

A 59-year-old woman becomes acutely short of breath two days after an acute myocardial infarction.

(a) List three possible causes for her shortness of breath
(3 marks)

(b) Give six investigations that you would perform immediately *(3 marks)*

(c) Briefly outline your management of the most likely diagnosis *(4 marks)*

Question 13

A 64-year-old man presents in the cardiology clinic with a two-year history of exertional chest pain and associated dyspnoea. More recently he has had three syncopal episodes whilst out walking his dog.

(a) (i) What is the cardiac valvular lesion causing his symptoms? *(1 mark)*
(ii) List two common causes of this lesion *(2 marks)*

(b) List three clinical signs that you would expect to find
(3 marks)

(c) Outline your investigations and further management
(4 marks)

Question 14

At a routine life assurance medical examination, a 47-year-old company director is found to have a blood pressure of 170/100 mmHg. No other significant clinical abnormalities are noted.

(a) List four investigations that you would perform

(2 marks)

(b) List four classes of drugs that you may consider using in this case, with an example of each *(4 marks)*

(c) Outline your management, assuming the diagnosis to be essential hypertension *(4 marks)*

Question 15

A 27-year-old sales representative presents to her GP with a three-month history of worsening headaches, malaise and lethargy. On examination her blood pressure is found to be 190/100 mmHg both lying and standing. There are no other cardiovascular abnormalities noted.

(a) List three endocrine disorders, other than diabetes, that may present with hypertension *(3 marks)*

(b) List three renal causes of hypertension *(3 marks)*

(c) Outline your further investigations *(4 marks)*

7

QUESTIONS

Haematology

Question 1

A 57-year-old office worker with treated hypertension visits his GP for routine follow-up. He is noted to be plethoric and a full blood count reveals his haemoglobin to be 21 g/dl.

(a) What is the name of this condition?   *(1 mark)*

(b) List four possible causes   *(4 marks)*

(c) What is (i) the treatment, and (ii) the prognosis, for the malignant form of this condition?   *(5 marks)*

Question 2

A 19-year-old man with known haemophilia B (Christmas disease) presents to the Emergency Department with a short history of increasing back pain. He is noted to be tachycardic and hypotensive. A CT scan shows a large retroperitoneal haematoma.

(a) List four possible emergency treatments to correct the coagulation defect *(4 marks)*

(b) What is the pathological basis of haemophilia B? *(3 marks)*

(c) List three complications of treatment *(3 marks)*

Question 3

You are called to see a 50-year-old woman who has undergone an elective hysterectomy for fibroids earlier in the day. She has suddenly become unwell about five minutes after starting to receive a blood transfusion. You diagnose an acute haemolytic transfusion reaction.

(a) List four clinical features and four laboratory tests (indicate expected results) that are indicative of this diagnosis *(4 marks)*

(b) What is the most common pathological basis of this reaction? *(1 mark)*

(c) Outline your management *(5 marks)*

Question 4

A 28-year-old man presents to the Emergency Department with a week's history of shortness of breath, fever and cough productive of small amounts of green sputum. Chest radiograph shows patchy shadowing throughout both hemithoraces. Full blood count is normal. He is started on intravenous amoxicillin. Three days later he is more dyspnoeic. The haematology lab technician telephones to say that the patient's latest haemoglobin is 5.3 g/dl and that the blood film shows evidence of haemolysis.

(a) What is the cause of the haemolytic anaemia?

(2 marks)

(b) List (i) three features of acute haemolysis on a blood film and (ii) three other haematological and/or biochemical tests, with expected results, that support your diagnosis *(3 marks)*

(c) Name five other causes of haemolytic anaemia

(5 marks)

Question 5

A 37-year-old woman presents to her GP with a nine-month history of progressive lethargy and malaise now associated with exertional dyspnoea. On examination she is clinically anaemic, but no other abnormalities are detected. Routine blood tests reveal her to have a microcytic anaemia.

(a) List three causes of a microcytic anaemia   *(3 marks)*

(b) List the further investigations that you would arrange   *(3 marks)*

(c) List four gastrointestinal and four extra-intestinal causes of this woman's anaemia   *(4 marks)*

Question 6

A 63-year-old woman presents to the medical outpatient department with a one-year history of increasing lethargy, weight gain and poor concentration. She also complains of dry hair and skin. Investigations confirm hypothyroidism and a macrocytic anaemia, with an MCV of 112 fl.

(a) Give two causes of the raised MCV in this case   *(2 marks)*

(b) Explain the autoimmune basis of her anaemia   *(3 marks)*

(c) Briefly outline your further management   *(5 marks)*

Question 7

A 9-year-old boy with known sickle cell disease presents to the Emergency Department with a two-day history of an upper respiratory tract infection associated with pain in his ribs, back and hips. He also complains of severe left upper quadrant pain.

(a) (i) Name two other haemoglobinopathies *(2 marks)*

(ii) What is the cause of his left upper quadrant pain? *(1 mark)*

(b) Outline your therapeutic management in this case *(3 marks)*

(c) In each of the categories listed below, give one pathological change associated with sickle cell disease: (i) skin, (ii) renal, (iii) biliary tree and (iv) bone *(4 marks)*

Question 8

A 27-year-old man presents to his GP with a two-month history of weight loss, lethargy and night sweats, now associated with generalised pruritus. On examination he has generalised lymphadenopathy and hepatosplenomegaly. He denies any risk factors for HIV disease.

(a) What is the diagnosis? *(1 mark)*

(b) List five investigations to confirm the diagnosis *(5 marks)*

(c) Outline the therapeutic options *(4 marks)*

Question 9

A 5-year-old girl presents to the Paediatric Outpatient Department with a three-week history of nose bleeds and a purpuric rash following an upper respiratory tract infection. The results of a full blood count organised by her GP are Hb 13.2 g/dl, WCC 7.8 × 10⁹/l, platelets 31 × 10⁹/l. The comment on the film reads 'no abnormal forms seen, grossly reduced platelet numbers'.

(a) What is the likely cause of her thrombocytopaenia?

(2 marks)

(b) List five other causes   *(5 marks)*

(c) Outline the therapeutic options in this case   *(3 marks)*

Question 10

A six-year-old boy with known trisomy 21 presents to the Paediatric Outpatient Department with a two-month history of malaise, lethargy and exertional dyspnoea, associated with easy bruising and several recent chest infections. On examination he has generalised lymphadenopathy and hepatosplenomegaly. He is clinically anaemic and has several large bruises.

(a) What is the underlying diagnosis and why is it particularly relevant in this case?   *(2 marks)*

(b) List three investigations to confirm the diagnosis

(3 marks)

(c) Briefly outline the management strategies used in this case   *(5 marks)*

Question 11

A 47-year-old woman presents to her GP with a two-month history of malaise, anorexia and an 8 kg weight loss, associated with left upper quadrant discomfort and occasional fever. On examination she is clinically anaemic and has a very enlarged spleen extending 15 cm below the left costal margin.

(a) (i) What is the likely haematological malignancy in this case?   *(1 mark)*

(ii) What is the chromosomal abnormality and the associated translocation?   *(1 mark)*

(b) List two other causes of 'massive' splenomegaly

(2 marks)

(c) (i) List three essential investigations that you would perform   *(3 marks)*

(ii) Outline your management   *(3 marks)*

Question 12

A 62-year-old retired man presents to the Emergency Department with a painful, bruised hip after a seemingly insignificant fall whilst out shopping. On examination he is clinically anaemic and has multiple bruises, particularly around his left hip, which is clinically fractured. This is confirmed on X-ray, which also reveals multiple lytic lesions throughout the pelvic and femoral bones.

(a) State the descriptive term for this type of fracture and the underlying diagnosis   *(2 marks)*

(b) List five investigations that you would perform
                                                          (5 marks)

(c) He has a corrected calcium of 4.2 mmol/l. Outline your treatment of this problem   *(3 marks)*

8

QUESTIONS

Dermatology

Question 1

A 47-year-old obese woman presents to her GP with deep jaundice and intense pruritus, associated with moderate right upper quadrant pain which has been worsening over the last seven days.

(a) What is the likely cause of her symptoms?   *(1 mark)*

(b) List four other disorders which may present with pruritus   *(4 marks)*

(c) Outline the general principles for treating pruritus   *(5 marks)*

Question 2

A 16-year-old schoolgirl presents to the Dermatology Outpatient Department with a two-week history of a red, tender, itchy rash over both palms, which coincided with her starting work at a hairdressers about one month before. In the past she has had a similar rash over the pinna of her ears, after having her ears pierced.

(a)   (i)   What is the name given to this type of rash?

(2 marks)

       (ii)   What is the likely cause in this case?   *(1 mark)*

(b)   List three other causes of this type of rash which may be relevant to this patient   *(3 marks)*

(c)   Briefly outline your management of this patient

(4 marks)

Question 3

A 7-year-old boy with known atopic eczema is admitted to hospital with an acute exacerbation of his rash, with a 'weeping' area around the face which looks infected. He also has local areas of lichenification affecting knees, elbows and neck.

(a)   What does the term 'lichenification' mean? Which surfaces of the body does atopic eczema characteristically affect?   *(3 marks)*

(b)   Give two disorders associated with atopic eczema. What is the immune-mediated abnormality?   *(3 marks)*

(c)   Outline your management in this case   *(4 marks)*

Question 4

A 29-year-old man with long-standing psoriasis presents to his GP with a worsening psoriatic rash, which in areas demonstrates the Koebner phenomenon. The GP arranges for his admission to hospital.

(a) What is the Koebner phenomenon? List two other disorders that demonstrate it *(3 marks)*

(b) List three sites, other than the extensor surfaces of the limbs, which may be affected by psoriasis *(3 marks)*

(c) List the therapeutic agents used in the treatment of psoriasis, giving a side-effect of each *(4 marks)*

Question 5

A 43-year-old woman presents to the Emergency Department with a one-week history of a dry cough, fever and general malaise, now associated with a severe blistering rash over the hands and feet, and affecting her eyes and mouth. On examination blistering and 'target' lesions are seen, and coarse crackles are heard in both lung fields.

(a) What is the name given to this rash and what is the eponymous syndrome that has developed? *(2 marks)*

(b) What is the likely cause of the rash in this woman? List three other causes *(4 marks)*

(c) Outline your investigations and management *(4 marks)*

Question 6

An 18-year-old woman presents to her GP with a seven-day history of fever, malaise and arthralgia associated with increasingly painful red, tender, round lesions over her shins. The symptoms have started since she began taking the oral contraceptive pill.

(a) What is the lesion that has developed on her shins?

(1 mark)

(b) List four other causes of this lesion *(4 marks)*

(c) Briefly outline your management *(5 marks)*

Question 7

A 72-year-old man presents to his GP with a blistering pruritic rash affecting his upper and lower limbs.

(a) Give three causes of a blistering rash in a man of this age *(3 marks)*

(b) List three discerning questions you would ask in the history to differentiate the possible causes *(3 marks)*

(c) The rash displays Nikolsky's sign
    (i) What is this sign and what is the underlying diagnosis? *(2 marks)*
    (ii) List two drugs used in its treatment *(2 marks)*

Question 8

A 29-year-old ginger-haired man presents to his GP with a new, large mole on his left upper arm. He has recently returned to the UK after living in South Africa for several years.

(a) List the features that would concern you about this 'mole' *(4 marks)*

(b) List three skin conditions associated with excessive sunlight exposure *(3 marks)*

(c) What are the therapeutic options if this was found to be a malignant melanoma? *(3 marks)*

Question 9

A 46-year-old man is sent to the Dermatology Outpatient Department with 'abnormal nails'. On examination he has onycholysis.

(a) Give two causes of onycholysis *(2 marks)*

(b) List two investigations for this patient *(2 marks)*

(c) What are the nail changes associated with the following disorders (i) iron deficiency, (ii) bronchiectasis, (iii) infective endocarditis, (iv) psoriasis, (v) chemotherapy, (vi) chronic liver disease *(6 marks)*

Question 10

A 37-year-old man presents to the Dermatology Outpatient Department with areas of depigmentation over his hands and chest. A clinical diagnosis of vitiligo is made.

(a) List three disorders that may be associated with depigmentation   *(3 marks)*

(b) List three disorders that are associated with vitiligo   *(3 marks)*

(c) List the essential investigations that you would perform   *(4 marks)*

9

QUESTIONS

Gastroenterology

Question 1

A 61-year-old publican presents to his GP with a six-week history of anorexia, unintentional weight loss and continuous epigastric pain that radiates to the back. On examination there is a palpable epigastric mass and an enlarged left supraclavicular lymph node. The clinical suspicion of gastric carcinoma is confirmed on investigation.

(a) State (i) the eponymous terms associated with the enlarged lymph node and (ii) four other common presenting symptoms of gastric carcinoma *(3 marks)*

(b) List (i) two investigations that are used in the initial diagnosis of gastric carcinoma and (ii) two investigations that are used in staging *(4 marks)*

(c) List three long-term complications of total gastrectomy *(3 marks)*

Question 2

A 40-year-old man complains of progressive difficulty in swallowing solids with a recent onset of vomiting following meals.

(a) How would you exclude a malignant stricture of the oesophagus?   *(3 marks)*

(b) Motility studies reveals abnormal peristalsis and sphincter spasm of the oesophagus
    (i) How is oesophageal function studied?   *(2 marks)*
    (ii) State the likely diagnosis and its underlying pathology   *(2 marks)*

(c) How would you treat this condition?   *(3 marks)*

Question 3

A 54-year-old woman presents with an 18-month history of heartburn, water brash and belching, with pain on swallowing.

(a) State your diagnosis and the underlying mechanism   *(3 marks)*

(b) How would you demonstrate acid reflux in this patient?   *(3 marks)*

(c) Outline the treatment of this condition   *(4 marks)*

Question 4

A 43-year-old male business executive is admitted through the Emergency Department with a three-day history of vomiting 'coffee ground' material and 18 months of progressive dyspeptic symptoms, which are partially relieved by antacids.

(a) State the probable clinical diagnosis *(2 marks)*

(b) State two investigations to confirm your diagnosis and the expected findings *(3 marks)*

(c) List the drugs and their therapeutic regimes used to cure this disease *(5 marks)*

Question 5

A 36-year-old woman is referred to the Gastroenterology Clinic with a nine-month history of weakness and weight loss associated with intermittent abdominal discomfort and distension. The stools are bulky pale and greasy.

(a) (i) List three malabsorption states that would fit her symptoms *(3 marks)*

(ii) State one investigation that would provide evidence for a definitive diagnosis, and list the possible findings *(2 marks)*

(b) The patient is placed on a gluten-free diet and obtains remission from her symptoms over the subsequent four months

(i) State the likely diagnosis *(2 marks)*

(ii) List the long-term complications of this condition *(3 marks)*

Question 6

A 26-year-old woman is seen at the Emergency Department with fever, malaise and bloody diarrhoea of six days' duration.

(a) List the possible diagnoses from her presentation
(3 marks)

(b) The patient is sent home on a course of antibiotics but her condition worsens, with abdominal pain and distension. She is febrile, with a pulse rate of 120 beats/min. Sigmoidoscope examination reveals pus and blood with mucosal ulceration
  (i)   State the diagnosis   *(1 mark)*
  (ii) List three life-threatening complications that may ensue if treatment is further delayed   *(3 marks)*

(c) How would you treat this patient?   *(3 marks)*

Question 7

A 40-year-old woman with long-standing chronic bowel symptoms is diagnosed as having Crohn's disease.

(a) (i)   List the main symptoms of this disease   *(2 marks)*
  (ii) List four extra-gastrointestinal manifestations of this disease   *(2 marks)*

(b) List the medical measures that are used to treat an acute exacerbation of this disease   *(3 marks)*

(c) State the indications for surgery in this disease
(3 marks)

Question 8

A 30-year-old man known to have an AIDS-related illness complains of nausea, intermittent diarrhoea and crampy abdominal pain of increasing severity. Clinical examination is suggestive of subacute bowel obstruction.

(a) (i) List two causes of bowel obstruction in AIDS
(2 marks)

(ii) List three opportunistic organisms that cause enteric infection in AIDS *(3 marks)*

(b) (i) How would you confirm bowel obstruction in this patient? *(2 marks)*

(ii) State the principles of treatment *(3 marks)*

Question 9

A 29-year-old overseas visitor complains of malaise, abdominal pain and diarrhoea with the passage of blood-stained mucus over an eight-week period. A diagnosis of amoebic colitis is made on sigmoidoscopic examination.

(a) (i) List the characteristic sigmoidoscopic findings in this disease *(3 marks)*

(ii) State how you would confirm the diagnosis
(2 marks)

(b) How would you screen for an amoebic liver abscess in this patient? *(2 marks)*

(c) List the drugs that are used to treat this disease *(3 marks)*

Question 10

A 40-year-old male alcoholic presents with a 20-month history of progressive central abdominal pain, anorexia and weight loss, and habituation to analgesic drugs. There is no history of jaundice.

(a) (i) State the probable clinical diagnosis *(1 mark)*

(ii) State one blood test to confirm this *(1 mark)*

(b) His stools were bulky, pale and offensive, and his fasting blood sugar level was moderately elevated. State the causes of these findings *(3 marks)*

(c) How would you treat this patient? *(5 marks)*

Question 11

A 46-year-old man complains of anorexia, malaise and weakness and is found to have a palpably enlarged, firm and irregular liver. A clinical diagnosis of cirrhosis is made.

(a) List other abdominal findings that are characteristic of this disease *(3 marks)*

(b) State four biochemical investigations that are used to assess the severity of this disease and their significance *(4 marks)*

(c) The patient subsequently has an episode of haematemesis. State its association with the underlying liver disease *(3 marks)*

Question 12

A 42-year-old man with a history of alcohol abuse complains of anorexia, malaise and weight loss over a three-month period. On examination he is found to have an enlarged, tender liver.

(a) Write a note on the clinical spectrum of alcoholic liver disease *(4 marks)*

(b) List the pathological features of the liver disease *(3 marks)*

(c) What are the prognostic indicators of this disease? *(3 marks)*

Question 13

Ten days after sustaining a severe head injury in a road traffic accident, a 26-year-old woman remains paralysed and ventilated in ITU. The nutrition team are asked to assess her with regard to her feeding requirements.

(a) What are the two forms of feeding that may be used? *(2 marks)*

(b) List four investigations or parameters that are used in the nutritional assessment *(4 marks)*

(c) List the factors that will determine what form of feeding you would recommend *(4 marks)*

Question 14

A 39-year-old man, who is a known chronic alcohol abuser, is brought into the Emergency Department in a state of haemodynamic shock. On arrival he vomits 500 ml of fresh blood.

(a) (i) What is the most likely cause of his haematemesis? *(1 mark)*

   (ii) List four other causes *(2 marks)*

(b) List the essential blood tests that you would perform *(3 marks)*

(c) Outline your management of this patient *(4 marks)*

Question 15

A 66-year-old man is admitted as an emergency, having vomited a considerable quantity of blood at home and feeling weak and faint.

(a) List the historical findings that may point to the cause of bleeding in the upper gastrointestinal tract *(4 marks)*

(b) State an investigation that provides an immediate diagnosis in this patient *(2 marks)*

(c) The cause of the bleeding is found to be an ulcerating tumour on the lesser curve of the stomach. List the investigations that you would perform and state the definitive treatment *(4 marks)*

10

Nephrology

Question 1

A 23–year-old woman is found on screening to have a blood pressure of 180/120 mmHg. Her serum creatinine rises substantially after she is started on an ACE inhibitor and a clinical diagnosis of renal artery stenosis is made.

(a) What is the usual pathological basis of renal artery stenosis in this age group? *(1 mark)*

(b) State the other serum biochemical abnormalities commonly seen in untreated renal artery stenosis and explain why they arise *(5 marks)*

(c) Outline your management of this patient *(4 marks)*

Question 2

A 32-year-old renal transplant recipient takes an immunosuppressive regimen of prednisolone, tacrolimus and mycophenolate mofetil. He is admitted to hospital with a urinary tract infection and septicaemia, which is treated successfully with ceftazidime and gentamicin. During this admission, his renal function deteriorates.

(a) List four candidate mechanisms for the deterioration in renal function *(2 marks)*

(b) State the mechanisms of action of prednisolone, tacrolimus and mycophenolate mofetil *(4 marks)*

(c) Provide two examples of other immunosuppressive agents used in renal transplantation and state a major adverse effect for each *(4 marks)*

Question 3

A 48-year-old man with end-stage renal failure, treated by haemodialysis, is reviewed in clinic. His haemoglobin is 9.2 g/dl.

(a) What are the probable mechanisms of his anaemia? *(3 marks)*

(b) Name four treatments for his anaemia *(4 marks)*

(c) List three chronic metabolic complications of haemodialysis-treated end-stage renal failure *(3 marks)*

Question 4

A 27-year-old woman presents to the Emergency Department with a two-day history of worsening left loin pain associated with fever, rigors and vomiting. It is her third such presentation in the past six months.

(a) What is the diagnosis? *(1 mark)*

(b) List four investigations that you would perform on admission *(4 marks)*

(c) Briefly outline your further management *(5 marks)*

Question 5

A 34-year-old woman is sent by her GP to the Medical Outpatient Department with a three-month history of poorly controlled hypertension, recurrent UTI and bilaterally palpable kidneys. A diagnosis of polycystic kidneys is confirmed on ultrasound scan.

(a) Give two other causes of bilaterally enlarged kidneys *(2 marks)*

(b) List five complications of polycystic kidneys *(5 marks)*

(c) Outline the therapeutic management *(3 marks)*

Question 6

A 15-year-old schoolboy presents to the Emergency Department with a ten-day history of increasing ankle and leg oedema. He has felt lethargic but denies any other systemic symptoms or fever. Investigations reveal a nephrotic syndrome, secondary to minimal change nephropathy.

(a) List the triad which characterises a nephrotic syndrome *(3 marks)*

(b) List the electron microscopic changes that characterise minimal change nephropathy *(2 marks)*

(c) List three investigations that you would perform, and outline your management of this patient *(5 marks)*

Question 7

A 35-year-old man is admitted to the Renal Unit for investigation of a nephrotic syndrome secondary to a suspected glomerulonephritis.

(a) List three causes of a nephrotic syndrome *(3 marks)*

(b) List three haematological and three non-haematological investigations that you would perform *(5 marks)*

(c) List two complications of the nephrotic syndrome *(2 marks)*

Question 8

A 29-year-old woman who has had poorly controlled insulin-dependent diabetes mellitus for the past 15 years presents to her GP with malaise and lethargy. She has recently been started on an ACE inhibitor for hypertension. Routine blood investigations arranged that day show FBC: Hb 7.9 g/dl, MCV 88 fl, MCH 35 pg, WCC 9.0·10⁹/l, platelets 310·10⁹/l; U&Es: Na 122 mmol/l, K 8.8 mmol/l, urea 37.1 mmol/l, creatinine 567 µmol/l

(a) List two diagnoses that may be made from these data
(2 marks)

(b) List three factors that contribute to her deranged renal function
(3 marks)

(c) Outline the management of hyperkalaemia   *(5 marks)*

Question 9

A 53-year-old woman with chronic rheumatoid arthritis is sent by her GP to the Renal Outpatient Department with worsening renal impairment and signs suggestive of a nephrotic syndrome.

(a) Give two possible causes of renal impairment in this patient
(2 marks)

(b) List three non-haematological investigations that you would perform
(3 marks)

(c) Briefly outline your management of this patient
(5 marks)

Question 10

A 29-year-old man presents to the Medical Outpatient Department with a three-week history of malaise, lethargy, arthralgia and myalgia, associated with a vasculitic rash. Examination reveals palpable nodules over several of his peripheral arteries and a blood pressure of 180/130 mmHg. Routine urinalysis shows large amounts of protein and some blood.

(a) What is the diagnosis? List two other causes of renal impairment and a vasculitic rash   *(3 marks)*

(b) List two immune markers that may occur in this group of disorders   *(2 marks)*

(c) List two other investigations that you would perform, and outline your therapeutic management   *(5 marks)*

Question 11

A 39-year-old man presents to his GP with a four-month history of malaise and lethargy, but no other specific systemic symptoms. Routine blood investigations are FBC: Hb 6.2 g/dl, MCV 81 fl, MCH 34 pg, WCC 9.0 × 10⁹/l, platelets 298 × 10⁹/l; U&Es: Na 132 mmol/l, K 5.8 mmol/l, urea 45.7 mmol/l, creatinine 890 μmol/l, glucose 7.4 mmol/l, corrected calcium 1.76 mmol/l, phosphate 3.7 mmol/l; LFTs: albumin 18g/l, AST 23IU/l, ALT 18 IU/L, alkaline phosphatase 211 IU/l.

(a) List three features that indicate this man has chronic renal failure *(3 marks)*

(b) List three tests/investigations that you could do in the GP surgery to elucidate the cause of his renal failure *(3 marks)*

(c) Briefly outline your management of the (i) anaemia, (ii) renal impairment, (iii) hypocalcaemia and (iv) hyperphosphataemia *(4 marks)*

Question 12

A 73-year-old woman is brought to the Emergency Department by ambulance, after being found unconscious at home by a neighbour.
On arrival she is confused, with a GCS of 12, and is haemodynamically stable. Initial investigations show FBC: Hb 14.2 g/dl, haematocrit 0.58,
WCC 31.2 × 10⁹/l (neutrophilia),
platelets 57 × 10⁹/l; U&Es: Na 152 mmol/l,
K 4.3 mmol/l, urea 35.7 mmol/l,
creatinine 290 µmol/l, glucose 38.5 mmol/l.

(a) List three diagnoses that can be inferred from these results *(3 marks)*

(b) List four further investigations that you would perform *(4 marks)*

(c) List two causes of prerenal, renal and postrenal impairment *(3 marks)*

Question 13

A five-year-old boy is admitted to hospital for investigation of a suspected renal tubular acidosis. Initial investigations by his GP show U&Es:
Na 134 mmol/l, K 3.1 mmol/l, chloride 114 mmol/l, bicarbonate 12 mmol/l, urea 4.1 mmol/l, creatinine 103 µmol/l.

(a) Calculate the anion gap, showing your calculations *(3 marks)*

(b) List the three types of renal tubular acidosis, with a cause for each *(3 marks)*

(c) List two diabetic causes of a high anion gap acidosis, outlining the general principles of your therapeutic management *(4 marks)*

11

Rheumatology and Connective Tissue Diseases

Question 1

A 71-year-old woman presents to her GP with a month-long history of difficulty climbing stairs, standing up from chairs and reaching into high shelves and cupboards. She has also developed a purple-red papular rash over her knuckles. Serum creatine kinase is grossly elevated. A diagnosis of dermatomyositis is made.

(a) State the eponymous name of the cutaneous sign
(1 mark)

(b) List (i) two confirmatory tests and (ii) two complications of this disease *(4 marks)*

(c) With which group of underlying disorders is this disease particularly associated? In the absence of leading signs or symptoms, list four appropriate further investigations *(5 marks)*

Question 2

A 37-year-old woman presents to her GP with a 6-month history of dry mouth, difficulty swallowing without water, itchy, red eyes and recurrent conjunctivitis. She is otherwise fit and well. Tests for anti-Ro and anti-La antibodies are positive.

(a) State the diagnosis and list four confirmatory tests

(4 marks)

(b) List six potential treatments *(3 marks)*

(c) Describe the prognostic importance of the positive antibody test for this patient *(3 marks)*

Question 3

An 80-year-old man presents to the Emergency Department with a one-day history of a painful left knee, without antecedent trauma. On examination he is febrile, hypotensive and mildly confused. The knee is hot, red, swollen and tender. A chronic venous ulcer is present on the right lower leg. Full blood count shows Hb 13.8 g/dl, MCV 90 fl, WCC 23 × 10^9/l, predominantly neutrophils, and platelets 400 × 10^9/l.

(a) State his two principal diagnoses and the differential for his knee pain *(3 marks)*

(b) What is the probable pathological cause of his presentation? *(2 marks)*

(c) Outline your management *(5 marks)*

Question 4

A 24-year-old radiographer presents to the Emergency Department with vaginal bleeding in the nineteenth week of her first pregnancy. In the past she suffered a deep venous thrombosis three weeks after starting a combined oral contraceptive pill. An ultrasound scan of the uterus shows an intrauterine death. She undergoes induction of labour. On the third day after delivery, she develops severe headache associated with papilloedema. MRI scan demonstrates a sagittal sinus thrombosis.

(a) What is the likely underlying diagnosis?   *(1 mark)*

(b) How would you confirm this?   *(1 mark)*

(c) List the characteristic features   *(3 marks)*

(d) Outline your management   *(5 marks)*

Question 5

A 29-year-old woman presents to the Medical Outpatient Department with a four-month history of painful, swollen proximal interphalangeal joints, associated with early morning stiffness, malaise and lethargy. X-rays of her hands show a symmetrical erosive arthropathy affecting the proximal interphalangeal joints.

(a) What is the likely cause of her arthropathy?   *(1 mark)*

(b) In the categories below, list an associated feature which may occur in this disorder: (i) eyes, (ii) skin, (iii) respiratory, (iv) cardiovascular and (v) renal
(5 marks)

(c) Outline your therapeutic management of this patient
(4 marks)

Question 6

An obese 67-year-old woman presents to her GP with a four-month history of increasing swelling, pain and stiffness in her right knee. She suffered a comminuted fracture of the distal right femur in a car accident, ten years previously.

(a) What is the likely cause of her arthritis?   *(1 mark)*

(b) List the radiological features that you would expect on an X-ray of her right knee joint   *(5 marks)*

(c) Briefly outline your therapeutic management of this patient   *(4 marks)*

Question 7

A 27-year-old woman presents in the Rheumatology Outpatient Department, with a six-week history of malaise and lethargy associated with painful joints in her hands and a worsening rash over her cheeks. On examination the joints of her hands are tender but otherwise normal. There is a 'butterfly' rash over her cheeks and vasculitic changes around her finger nails.

(a) What is the underlying diagnosis?   *(1 mark)*

(b) List three immune markers that may occur in this disorder   *(3 marks)*

(c) In each of the categories below, list one pathological feature that may occur: (i) skin, (ii) vascular, (iii) renal, (iv) neurological, (v) haematological and (vi) musculoskeletal   *(6 marks)*

Question 8

A 39-year-old woman presents to her GP with a one-year history of pain in her fingers and toes associated with 'blanching' on exposure to the cold. She also complains of tightness and swelling of the fingers and, more recently, dysphagia with solids.

(a) What is the term used to describe the changes she experiences in the cold? *(1 mark)*

(b) This disorder was previously called the CREST syndrome. What are the components of the syndrome and what is it now called? *(4 marks)*

(c) Outline your therapeutic management of this patient *(5 marks)*

Question 9

A 47-year-old man presents to his GP with an acutely hot, tender and swollen interphalangeal joint of his left big toe. He is otherwise systemically well.

(a) What is the likely cause of his monoarthritis? *(1 mark)*

(b) List three investigations that would help confirm the diagnosis *(3 marks)*

(c) List three risk factors for developing this condition, and three drugs that you might use in this man's treatment, with a side-effect of each *(6 marks)*

Question 10

A 71-year-old woman presents to her GP with a four-week history of stiffness and pain in her shoulders and thighs, particularly on waking in the morning. Routine investigations reveal an ESR of 105.

(a) What is the likely cause of her symptoms and the associated arteritis? *(2 marks)*

(b) Give two other musculoskeletal conditions that may cause an ESR over 100 *(2 marks)*

(c) With regard to the arteritis:
  (i) List one investigation that confirms the diagnosis *(2 marks)*
  (ii) Which essential treatment must be instituted immediately? *(1 mark)*
  (iii) List three presenting symptoms *(3 marks)*

Question 11

A 41-year-old man presents to the Medical Outpatient Department with a six-month history of malaise and weight loss associated with a bloody nasal discharge, a chronic dry cough, episodic haemoptysis and exertional dyspnoea. On examination he has a vasculitic rash over his fingers and toes and coarse crackles are heard throughout both lung fields. Routine urinalysis shows large amounts of blood and protein in the urine.

(a) State the diagnosis, and the classical triad which forms the basis of this diagnosis   *(4 marks)*

(b) List two other causes of a vasculitic rash   *(2 marks)*

(c) List three investigations that you would perform, and name the drug that forms the basis of therapy
(4 marks)

Question 12

A 55-year-old woman, who had had a hysterectomy and bilateral salpingo-oophorectomy at the age of 34, presents to her GP with severe lumbar back pain. Routine blood tests are unremarkable, but X-rays of her lumbar spine show 'gross osteopenia and vertebral collapse at L2/L3'.

(a) What is the likely cause of her vertebral collapse?

(1 mark)

(b) (i) List three risk factors for developing this condition

(3 marks)

(ii) List the therapeutic agents that you would use in this case *(3 marks)*

(c) Outline the advice that you would give her 22-year-old daughter with regard to prophylaxis *(3 marks)*

Question 13

A 77-year-old man with known Paget's disease of the bone presents to the Emergency Department with a four-week history of increasing pain in his right hip and lumbar spine. He is now unable to bear weight.

(a) What is the pathological basis of Paget's bone disease?

(2 marks)

(b) List three investigations that you would perform to confirm the diagnosis *(3 marks)*

(c) List three complications of Paget's bone disease, and briefly outline your therapeutic management

(5 marks)

Question 14

A 63-year-old man with known ankylosing spondylitis presents to his GP with worsening mobility and lumbar back pain. On examination he has severely restricted lumbar and cervical spine movement and mild vertebral tenderness over the lumbosacral spine.

(a) What is the HLA association of this disorder? List two other diseases that are linked to this HLA serotype
(3 marks)

(b) List the radiological features that may be present on an X-ray of this man's lumbosacral spine *(3 marks)*

(c) In the categories below, list one pathological feature that may occur in this disorder (i) eyes, (ii) cardiac, (iii) respiratory, (iv) neurological *(4 marks)*

Question 15

A 26-year-old man returns from a business trip in Bangkok with a one-week history of a painful urethral discharge associated with gritty, painful red eyes and a hot swollen left knee. In the last 24 hours he has also developed ulceration in his mouth and on the glans penis.

(a) State the eponymous name given to the disorder described above, and the triad of symptoms which define it *(2 marks)*

(b) List three organisms that may precipitate it *(3 marks)*

(c) Briefly outline your investigations and therapeutic management *(5 marks)*

Psychiatry

Question 1

A 20-year-old man is brought to hospital by police having been found wandering along the central reservation of the M4 on a Friday afternoon. He had become agitated in the police van and a police surgeon administered an intramuscular dose of haloperidol prior to transfer to hospital. Now calmer, the patient tells you he has been treated for schizophrenia for the last 18 months with clozapine.

(a) Clozapine belongs to which class of drug?   *(1 mark)*

(b) State (i) its most prominent serious adverse effect and (ii) the measures required in detecting its onset

(4 marks)

(c) Suggest five possible mechanisms to explain the deterioration in this patient's mental illness   *(5 marks)*

Question 2

A 39-year-old man reluctantly attends his GP with his wife. She feels that his alcohol intake is becoming a problem, but he cannot see 'the harm of the odd drink here and there'.

(a) What are the four elements of the CAGE questionnaire?   *(4 marks)*

(b) List two screening investigations to assess this man's alcohol intake   *(2 marks)*

(c) Outline your management of this patient   *(4 marks)*

Question 3

A 72-year-old man, whose wife recently died in a road traffic accident, is found deeply unconscious in bed, by his neighbour. On the bedside table there is a long suicide note, accompanied by an empty bottle of pills.

(a) List three features of the history that imply this was a serious suicide attempt   *(3 marks)*

(b) List three other factors that are used to determine suicidal intent   *(3 marks)*

(c) Briefly outline your management in this case   *(4 marks)*

Question 4

A 19-year-old student visits her college GP with a four-month history of amenorrhoea. She denies being pregnant and has put it down to the stress of the course. The GP cannot help noticing that she is extremely thin, and on further questioning she does admit to eating 'very infrequently' recently.

(a) What is the likely diagnosis? List two criteria used to make this diagnosis *(3 marks)*

(b) The student is 1.6 metres tall and weighs 30 kg. Calculate her BMI, showing your calculations *(3 marks)*

(c) List three investigations that you would perform, and briefly outline your management *(4 marks)*

Question 5

A 29-year-old known heroin addict is brought into to the Emergency Department unconscious, with shallow respiration and a thready pulse.

(a) (i) What is the diagnosis, and the immediate management? *(3 marks)*
(ii) Which other physical sign will confirm the diagnosis? *(1 mark)*

(b) List two routes of administration that are commonly used by heroin addicts *(2 marks)*

(c) In the categories below, list one symptom or sign that may be exhibited on the withdrawal of heroin
(i) neurological, (ii) psychological,
(iii) gastrointestinal and (iv) dermatological *(4 marks)*

Question 6

A GP is called to see a 31-year-old woman, who has recently lost her six-year-old daughter, who died of leukaemia. She has not been out since the funeral one month ago, and her husband is very worried that she has completely withdrawn into herself.

(a) What is the underlying diagnosis? List two other features that you would specifically try to elicit in the history *(3 marks)*

(b) List two non-pharmacological therapies that may be employed *(2 marks)*

(c) List the four main classes of antidepressants, with an example and a side-effect of each class *(5 marks)*

Question 7

A 26-year-old unemployed man is brought into the Emergency Department by the police, who found him wandering naked in the local park. They say he was screaming at some men who were 'trying to kill him' when, in fact, he was alone. Examination and investigations are unremarkable and he is referred to the psychiatrist with a clinical diagnosis of schizophrenia.

(a) List two first rank symptoms of schizophrenia *(2 marks)*

(b) List two presenting and two premorbid features that indicate a poor prognosis in schizophrenia *(4 marks)*

(c) Briefly outline your therapeutic management *(4 marks)*

Question 8

A 31-year-old man is brought to the psychiatric outpatient department by his wife, with a three-month history of working 20 hours per day whilst sleeping for only two to three hours. He claims he has become the managing director of his accountancy firm when, in fact, he has just been made redundant. She says he has also become sexually demanding. He was treated for depression by his GP one year previously.

(a) What are the terms that are used to describe his present condition and the underlying condition?　*(3 marks)*

(b) List three presenting features of this disorder in the history　*(3 marks)*

(c) List two drugs used in the treatment of this disorder and a side-effect of each　*(4 marks)*

Question 9

A 27-year-old man is referred by his lawyer to see a psychiatrist for assessment. He is a habitual criminal, with multiple convictions for violent crime. He has been married three times, each ending in divorce, after he was violent towards his family. He has never had a permanent job and is at present on remand, after fatally stabbing a man in a fight.

(a) What is the term used to describe this man's behavioural disorder? *(2 marks)*

(b) Define what is meant by a personality disorder, listing three other examples *(5 marks)*

(c) List the factors that may have influenced the development of this type of personality *(3 marks)*

Question 10

A 32-year-old man is referred to the Psychiatric Outpatient Department by his GP with a six-month history of washing his hands up to 50 times per day, to the point where his hands have become ulcerated and raw.

(a) What is the term used to describe this condition? *(2 marks)*

(b) Define the term neurosis, giving two examples *(4 marks)*

(c) Briefly outline your management *(4 marks)*

13

Care of the Elderly

Question 1

A 76-year-old man with vascular dementia is noted by his wife, with whom he still lives at home, to have lost weight. She also notices blood in his stools when she helps him with toileting. They walk to their GPs surgery together, where a clinical diagnosis of a rectal tumour is made, based on a digital rectal examination.

(a) Outline the relevant ethical issues regarding further investigation   (6 marks)

(b) He is seen in clinic by a consultant colorectal surgeon. The digital rectal examination is repeated, briefly, but the patient is unwilling to lie still. A decision is made to admit him for investigation, including examination under anaesthesia. Outline the criteria by which the patient's capacity to consent to this procedure should be judged   (4 marks)

Question 2

An 88-year-old woman presents to her GP with a two-month history of increased bowel frequency and of passing loose stools, that contain mucus and blood. She also complains of fatigue, 8 kg weight loss and intermittent, colicky lower abdominal pain.

(a) State (i) the most likely diagnosis and (ii) three differential diagnoses   *(4 marks)*

(b) List four signs that would support the most likely diagnosis   *(2 marks)*

(c) Outline your investigation strategy   *(4 marks)*

Question 3

An 94-year-old woman develops faecal incontinence whilst recuperating in hospital from surgery for a fractured neck of femur. Digital rectal examination reveals the presence of hard stool in the rectum.

(a) What is the cause of the faecal incontinence?   *(2 marks)*

(b) Outline your management   *(4 marks)*

(c) List eight other causes of faecal incontinence   *(4 marks)*

Question 4

A 77-year-old man presents in the Outpatient Department with his wife, who gives a six-month history of a stepwise progressive deterioration in his memory, associated with worsening confusion and urinary incontinence. He has had two previous strokes and has been hypertensive for the past 15 years.

(a) What is the diagnosis? *(1 mark)*

(b) List ten questions you would use to assess the degree of this man's cognitive impairment *(5 marks)*

(c) List the important features that you would elicit in the social history and the members of the multidisciplinary team you would employ to achieve plans to keep this man at home *(4 marks)*

Question 5

An 83-year-old woman who is normally fit and well is brought to the Emergency Department, having been found lying confused on the bedroom floor by her neighbours. On examination, she has a GCS of 13, her capillary blood glucose is above the range of the meter and she is pyrexial with an axillary temperature of 38.0°C. She is in atrial fibrillation with a fast ventricular response, and has coarse crackles at the right lung base. Her mental test score is 3/10, but there is no focal neurological deficit.

(a) Give one possible cause for her admission *(1 mark)*

(b) List five haematological and five non-haematological investigations that you would perform *(5 marks)*

(c) Outline your therapeutic management *(4 marks)*

Question 6

An 86-year-old woman presents to the Outpatient Department with a three-month history of recurrent falls. She is being treated with a loop diuretic and an ACEI for heart failure and low-dose aspirin for ischaemic heart disease. She has recently been started on digoxin for atrial fibrillation.

(a) Give three possible causes for this woman's falls

(3 marks)

(b) List three investigations that you would perform

(3 marks)

(c) List a side-effect of each of the medications she is taking   *(4 marks)*

Question 7

A 79-year-old woman with a three-year history of mild to moderate dementia presents to the outpatient department with a two-month history of worsening urinary incontinence.

(a) List three possible causes for her incontinence

(3 marks)

(b) List three investigations that you would perform

(3 marks)

(c) Outline the therapeutic options   *(4 marks)*

Question 8

An 81-year-old woman is recovering in hospital two weeks after surgery on a fractured right neck of femur. The orthopaedic surgeon has requested a review, to help with her recovery.

(a) List three possible causes for her slow progress

(3 marks)

(b) List six investigations that you would request

(3 marks)

(c) Outline your management plan for this woman's rehabilitation *(4 marks)*

Question 9

An 84-year-old man is brought into the Emergency Department by ambulance, after having been found unconscious at home. On examination he has a rectal temperature of 31°C, a GCS of 5 and a capillary blood glucose of 9.8 mmol/l. There is no focal neurological deficit, and he has flexor plantar responses. Cardiovascular examination reveals an irregular pulse, with a rate of 30 beats/minute, but the blood pressure is 110/70 mmHg. The rest of the clinical examination is normal.

(a) What is the cause of this man's coma?
List three predisposing factors *(3 marks)*

(b) List six essential investigations that you would perform *(3 marks)*

(c) Outline your management *(4 marks)*

Question 10

A 91-year-old man is admitted to hospital with a three-month history of worsening prostatism, associated with lumbar back and rib pain. Subsequent investigation reveals him to have disseminated prostatic carcinoma with bony metastases.

(a) List the major symptoms you would address in this case *(3 marks)*

(b) List six drugs that may be required in this man's treatment *(3 marks)*

(c) Outline your management once the diagnosis has been confirmed *(4 marks)*

PART TWO

SAQ Model Answers and Comments

Infectious Diseases

Answer 1

(a) Leptospirosis; *Leptospira interrogans*   *(3 marks)*

(b) Doxycycline 100 mg po bd for one week
Benzylpenicillin 900–1200 mg IV six-hourly for
one week   *(2 marks)*

(c) Oliguria/anuria/uraemia/renal failure
Jaundice/hepatomegaly/hepatic tenderness
Purpura/petechiae/gum bleeding/major internal
haemorrhage
Meningitis/encephalitis/encephalopathy
Death   *(5 marks)*

Comment

Leptospirosis occurs throughout the world but is particularly prevalent in the tropics. *Leptospira interrogans* is shed in mammalian urine and survives best in warm fresh water. In the UK, recreational exposure to fresh water (eg canoeing, sailing) is the major cause of infection. After an incubation period ranging from a few days to four weeks, the disease presents with fever, rigors, myalgia and headache. Conjunctival suffusion commonly occurs after two to three days. In many cases the symptoms resolve after about a week, sometimes returning briefly a few days later. Meningitis, renal impairment or bleeding at mucosal surfaces may occur but the majority of infections are probably unrecognised clinically. However, a small proportion of patients progress to develop Weil's disease, a life-threatening manifestation of leptospirosis in which jaundice occurs about one week after the onset of symptoms. Renal failure and major haemorrhage are characteristic features of Weil's disease and it is these, rather than liver failure, that are responsible for mortality. Treatment consists of antibiotics and supportive measures, particularly ensuring adequate hydration. If treatment is started sufficiently early, the prognosis is excellent.

Answer 2

(a) (i)   Lyme disease/Lyme borreliosis
   (ii) *Borrelia burgdorferi*
   (iii) *Ixodes* tick
   (iv) Erythema migrans   *(4 marks)*

(b) Carditis causing atrioventricular block
   VIIth nerve palsy
   Meningitis
   Encephalomyelitis
   Peripheral neuropathy
   Acrodermatitis chronica atrophicans
   Borrelial lymphocytoma   *(4 marks)*

(c) Doxycycline
   Amoxicillin   *(2 marks)*

Comment

Lyme disease, or Lyme borreliosis, is named after the town of Lyme, Connecticut, USA, where it was first recognised. It results from infection by the *Borrelia burgdorferi* spirochaete, the vector for which is the *Ixodes* tick. A characteristic rash, known as erythema migrans, starts at the site of the tick bite, usually between one and two weeks after detachment of the tick. An erythematous macule spreads slowly out from the centre, which often clears to give a 'target' appearance. In untreated cases, the rash usually resolves after about a month. Ticks may sometimes be found attached at the site of the bite; if removed within 36 hours of initial attachment, the risk of spirochaete transmission is very low.

Joint involvement presents as an intermittent mono- or oligoarthritis, often migratory but almost invariably affecting the knee at some point. Articular signs and symptoms usually resolve promptly with appropriate antibiotics, with the addition of a NSAID if necessary. A fortnight's course of oral doxycycline or amoxicillin is sufficient to treat uncomplicated erythema migrans, VIIth nerve palsy or oligoarthritis. Intravenous antibiotics, usually ceftriaxone or benzylpenicillin, are reserved for cases of meningitis or heart block.

Answer 3

(a) *Pneumocystis carinii* pneumonia
Mycobacterium tuberculosis
Other bacterial pneumonia, eg *Streptococcus pneumoniae*
Fungal infiltration, eg *Aspergillus* spp
Bronchiolitis obliterans   *(3 marks)*

(b) History and examination
Arterial blood gases
Pulse oximetry before and after exercise
Chest X-ray
Sputum, induced if necessary, for microscopy, culture and sensitivity
Bronchoscopy and bronchoalveolar lavage   *(4 marks)*

(c) Oxygen therapy
Co-trimoxazole (high dose) for three weeks
Glucocorticoids for first week (if arterial $<p_a(O_2)$ 9.3 kPa)
Pentamidine for patients allergic to co-trimoxazole
Prophylaxis, eg low-dose co-trimoxazole, to continue indefinitely   *(3 marks)*

Comment

Effective prophylaxis, as well as highly active antiretroviral therapy, (for HIV disease) has rendered *Pneumocystis carinii* pneumonia much less common than in the latter part of the twentieth century. Nevertheless, it remains one of the characteristic late complications of HIV disease. The clinical features

CHAPTER 1 – ANSWERS

usually include gradually increasing breathlessness, a dry cough, fever and malaise. Chest signs are often minimal but arterial oxygen desaturation, if not present at rest, is provoked by exercise, an observation that may be demonstrated conveniently using pulse oximetry. The characteristic radiographic appearance is of bilateral perihilar shadowing. Definitive diagnosis may require bronchoscopy and bronchoalveolar lavage but this may sometimes be avoided using induced sputum collection. Cysts and trophozoites are demonstrated on microscopy of the sputum. After successful treatment, prophylaxis should be continued indefinitely, although it may be discontinued if the immune system responds to antiretroviral therapy.

Answer 4

(a) Ophthalmoscopy (for papilloedema and retinal involvement in infection)
Examination for evidence of meningeal irritation
Cranial nerve examination   *(1 mark)*

(b) (i) Cerebral toxoplasmosis with surrounding oedema causing raised intracranial pressure
(ii) Sulfadiazine (or clindamycin) with pyrimethamine and highly active antiretroviral therapy   *(4 marks)*

(c) Cryptococcal meningitis
HIV encephalopathy
CMV encephalitis
Progressive multifocal leukoencephalopathy
Non-Hodgkin's lymphoma   *(5 marks)*

Comment

This patient's presentation suggests an intracerebral space-occupying lesion of septic origin. The most common cause of this in late HIV disease is *Toxoplasma gondii*. CT scanning of the brain with contrast typically reveals multiple ring-enhancing lesions with surrounding oedema. The diagnosis is usually made on the basis of clinical findings and radiographic appearances, with brain biopsy only being considered if the patient fails to respond to treatment. The differential includes cerebral lymphoma and abscesses caused by other organisms, eg tuberculosis.

Cerebral toxoplasmosis is treated effectively by a combination of either sulfadiazine or clindamycin with pyrimethamine. Recurrence is common so treatment is continued indefinitely, or until an adequate immune recovery occurs with highly active antiretroviral therapy.

Answer 5

(a) Chronic hepatitis B or C virus infection *(1 mark)*

(b) Transplacentally
Blood borne: sexual, blood transfusion, intravenous drug user (IVDU), tattooing *(3 marks)*

(c) Investigations:
  LFTs and clotting screen
  Hepatitis B and C serology
  Alpha fetoprotein
  US scan of the liver
  Liver biopsy
Therapeutic management:
  Immunomodulatory therapy:
    pegylated interferon alfa
  Nucleoside analogues:
    lamivudine, adefovir dipivoxil (for HBV)
    ribavirin (for HCV)
  Exclude the development of hepatocellular carcinoma (HCC)
  Screen family members and sexual contacts
  (6 marks)

Comment

Viral hepatitis is a common cause of chronic liver disease, particularly in endemic areas such as South East Asia. It is the major aetiological risk factor in the development of primary hepatocellular carcinoma. HBV infection is caused by a DNA virus, which has three main antigenic components: the surface protein, HBs antigen; the core protein, HBc antigen; and a soluble protein produced from the core gene, HBe antigen. These all give rise to antibody responses, the significances of which are summarised below.

	Antigen	**Antibody**
HBs	Marker of viral replication, it is found in acute, chronic and carrier states	Marker of immunity, it shows previous exposure to the virus or vaccination
HBc	It is not usually seen in the blood and has no clinical significance	There are two antibody responses, IgM and IgG. IgM is a marker of ongoing viral replication
HBe	Marker of infectivity, its persistence in the plasma signifies a chronic or carrier state, with a high risk of infectivity	This is a marker of low infectivity risk

At-risk groups, such as health-care workers, should be vaccinated. Secondary prevention with hyperimmune serum globulin, containing anti-HBs antibody, can also be given in cases of accidental exposure, eg needle stick injury. Antiviral treatment rarely eradicates the virus completely but may achieve seroconversion from HBe antigen to HBe antibody positive, reducing infectivity. It may also reverse cirrhotic changes. In patients developing hepatocellular carcinoma, surgical resection or liver transplantation may be considered, although in localised disease, radiological embolisation of the tumour now offers a less invasive approach. Chemotherapy using adriamycin is used as an adjunct.

Answer 6

(a) Meningitis
Neisseria meningitidis
Streptococcus pneumoniae
Haemophilus influenzae   *(3 marks)*

(b) Blood tests: FBC, U&Es, glucose, clotting screen to
include D-dimer and FDPs, blood cultures
CT head scan: to exclude significantly raised
intracranial pressure
Lumbar puncture: MC+S, protein and glucose
ASO titre
Throat swab
CXR   *(3 marks)*

(c) The patient should be nursed in a darkened,
quiet room
Intravenous access, IV fluids
Analgesia and antiemetics
Start empirical IV antibiotic therapy
In children (<15 years old) dexamethasone
Correction of clotting abnormalities using FFP
and platelets
Contact tracing and chemoprophylaxis   *(4 marks)*

Comment

Bacterial meningitis remains a serious infection with a mortality of
10%–50%, depending on the causative organism. It is essential
therefore to have a low threshold of suspicion and to start empirical
intravenous antibiotic treatment whenever the diagnosis is being
considered. The causative organisms tend to be age specific:

Neonates: *E. coli*, *Listeria*, group B streptococci

Children (<15 years): *Neisseria meningitidis*, *Streptococcus
pneumoniae*, *Haemophilus influenzae*

Adults: similar to children but also *Staphylococcus aureus*, *E. coli*
and *Listeria*

If delays are envisaged at any point in the management then empirical IV antibiotic therapy should be given using benzylpenicillin, cefotaxime, ceftazidime, or ceftriaxone. Chloramphenicol is still used in some cases, but it is highly toxic and must be used with caution. In children under the age of 15, intravenous or oral dexamethasone should be given, as this reduces the postmeningitic complications, in particular deafness and residual cerebral damage. Symptomatic relief with appropriate analgesia, intravenous fluids and anti-emetics are important in all cases. In severe cases with septicaemic shock, DIC and multi-organ failure the patient will require intensive care with inotrope support and, occasionally, renal dialysis.

Answer 7

(a) *Mycobacterium tuberculosis* *(1 mark)*

(b) Blood cultures: MC+S, AAFBs
Sputum for MC+S, AAFBs
Stool culture
CXR
Barium meal and follow-through
laparoscopic biopsy of affected bowel *(5 marks)*

(c) Rifampicin: derangement of LFTs, causes secretions, eg urine, to turn red
Isoniazid: peripheral neuropathy (therefore given with pyridoxine)
Pyrazinamide: hepatotoxic
Streptomycin: ototoxic
Ethambutol: optic neuritis *(4 marks)*

Comment

This woman has developed disseminated tuberculosis infection (TB), involving the lungs and terminal ileum. Diagnosis may be inferred by chest X-ray and barium follow-through appearances, and confirmed by the presence of alcohol and acid fast bacilli (AAFB) in sputum, blood and biopsy specimens. In cases where the small bowel is affected the patient may present with a clinical picture similar to that of terminal ileal Crohn's disease. However, this is rare in people of the Indian subcontinent and an empirical trial of antituberculous treatment should be started. As in any disorder presenting with chronic diarrhoea, a full nutritional assessment of the patient should be made, and possible nutritional support instituted. Management of any patient with TB should include a full course of antituberculous treatment, and contact tracing. Those in close contact with the patient should be tested for the disease by Mantoux testing and chest X-ray. Those tested negative should then receive BCG inoculation. Patients should receive regular follow-up to ensure compliance and treatment success, as well as patient wellbeing. Ideally this should be directed from a centre and team dedicated to TB treatment. Non-compliance has led to the emergence of resistant strains of TB (MDRTB), particularly in the USA.

Most patients in the UK with pulmonary TB are prescribed rifampicin and isoniazid (with pyridoxine) for six months, supplemented for the first two months with pyrazinamide and ethambutol (streptomycin is reserved for resistant cases). In extrapulmonary TB, the regimen is given for one year, with each period above being doubled.

Answer 8

(a) *Plasmodium vivax, Plasmodium ovale* – chloroquine and primaquine
Plasmodium falciparum – quinine and pyrimethamine with sulfadoxine (Fansidar)
Plasmodium malariae–chloroquine   *(3 marks)*

(b) Blood tests: FBC, U&Es, glucose, LFTs, clotting screen
Thick and thin blood films for malaria
Blood cultures
MSU
CXR
Stool cultures for ovum, parasites and cysts   *(3 marks)*

(c)   Primary prophylaxis against being bitten by mosquitoes
      Mosquito net over the bed, mosquito repellent,
      wear pyjama trousers and sleeves at night
      Full course of antimalarial tablets, stressing the
      need for full compliance
      Ensure all vaccinations, including typhoid, tetanus,
      polio, hepatitis A and B, are up to date   *(4 marks)*

Comment

Malaria remains one of the commonest infectious causes of
mortality worldwide, accounting for over a million deaths per year.
It is endemic in Central and South America, sub-Saharan Africa,
the Middle East, the Indian subcontinent and South East Asia. In
these areas, there is a high prevalence of haemoglobinopathies
amongst the local population and this confers a natural resistance
to the disease. So-called benign malaria is caused by three species of
the parasite, *Plasmodium vivax, Plasmodium ovale* and *Plasmodium
malariae*. Although they tend to run a benign course, these
parasites are responsible for chronic disease due to the dormant
hepatic phase in their life cycle. This varies between months and
years, and gives rise to hepatomegaly, 'giant' splenomegaly and
chronic renal failure. They are invariably sensitive to chloroquine
(reported resistance is limited principally to Papua New Guinea)
and, if identified in blood films, the hepatic phase should be
covered for with primaquine. Falciparum malaria is termed the
'malignant' malaria, is present in sub-saharan Africa, and is
responsible for the majority of the associated mortality. Death is
caused by cerebral involvement, DIC and multi-organ failure.
There may be acute renal tubular necrosis or a glomerulonephritis
causing renal failure and, commonly, there is pulmonary oedema
and secondary bronchopneumonia, which is often the terminal
event. In all cases of suspected malaria, falciparum disease must
always be covered for, until there is definite species identification.
The patient should be started immediately on quinine either orally,
or, if severely unwell or cerebral involvement is suspected,
intravenously. Other drugs used in the treatment of falciparum
disease include Fansidar® and halofantrine.

Answer 9

(a) Infectious mononucleosis caused by
Epstein–Barr virus (EBV)
Cytomegalovirus (CMV)
Toxoplasmosis
HIV
Lymphoma *(3 marks)*

(b) FBC with differential, blood film and monospot test
Paul–Bunnell test
Specific antibody tests for EBV, CMV, toxoplasmosis
Throat swab
ASO titre
Lymph node biopsy *(5 marks)*

(c) Most of the causes are self-limiting, requiring
symptomatic relief only, ie analgesia for the
pharyngitis, regular paracetamol for pyrexia
and fluids

Severe cases may require hospitalisation and
specific treatment, eg steroids in EBV infection
(2 marks)

Comment

EBV, CMV and toxoplasmosis may all present in a similar clinical
manner, with pharyngitis, lymphadenopathy and splenomegaly
associated with a low-grade fever and flu-like symptoms. Infectious
mononucleosis is caused by the Epstein–Barr virus and most
commonly presents in adolescents and young adults. It is usually a
self-limiting disorder, requiring no specific treatment. In more severe
cases the use of steroids is advocated. Common sequelae include:

- Meningitis, encephalitis
- Myocarditis
- Hepatitis
- Splenomegaly – more rarely splenic rupture
- Guillain–Barré syndrome
- Haemolytic anaemia and thrombocytopaenia

CHAPTER 1 – ANSWERS

EBV infection is strongly linked to the development of Burkitt's lymphoma. CMV infection is particularly prevalent in immunocompromised patients, being common in HIV-positive and transplant patients. In these patients it may produce a severe illness, similar to EBV infection, and should be treated with intravenous ganciclovir. It is differentiated from EBV infection by specific IgG and IgM antibodies, and the presence of intranuclear 'owl eyes' inclusions in tissue biopsy samples. Toxoplasmosis is a protozoan infection, caused by *Toxoplasma gondii*. Humans act as the intermediate host in its life cycle. The infection is usually carried by cats which are infected by killing and eating infected mice and birds. It is usually a self-limiting disorder, but may present in the immunocompromised as a severe febrile illness, involving the liver, spleen, central nervous system and heart. This is treated with a combination of pyrimethamine and sulphadiazine. Steroids are used in ocular disease. The infection may also be acquired transplacentally, where it produces a chronic central nervous system disorder, characterised by hydrocephalus, cerebral calcification, chorioretinitis and seizures, classically known as the syndrome of Savin.

Answer 10

(a) (i) Chancre of primary syphilis or
gonorrhoea *(1 mark)*

(ii) *Neisseria gonorrhoeae*
Treponema pallidum *(2 marks)*

(b) Other sexually acquired infections – HBV and HCV infection
HIV
Chlamydial NSU
Genital and oral HSV infection
Anal and genital warts *(3 marks)*

(c) Urethral swab – MC+S, wet preparation for
Trichomonas
Syphilis serology
HIV test, with pretest counselling
Treatment – procaine penicillin by intramuscular
injection
If allergic to penicillin – tetracycline or
erythromycin
Tracing of sexual contacts
Education about sexual behaviour   *(4 marks)*

Comment

Syphilis is a sexually transmitted disease, caused by the spirochaete
Treponema pallidum. Except for a slight rise in the early 1970s, the
incidence of the infection fell consistently through the twentieth
century. Sadly this trend has now been reversed with significant
rises over the last 5 years. This is thought to be due to young
people ignoring the risks of unprotected sexual intercourse. It is
divided into primary, secondary and tertiary infection by various
clinical manifestations. The duration of each phase varies between
weeks and years. Syphilis serological tests indicate the stage and
infectivity of the disease, and are explained below.

	VDRL	TPHA	FTA
Primary–early	–	–	+
Primary–late	+	+	+
Secondary	Rising titres	+	+
Tertiary	Rising titres	+	+

The *Treponema pallidum* haemagglutination assay (TPHA), and
the fluorescent *Treponema* antibodies-absorbed test (FTA) are
highly specific markers of syphilitic infection, but they will always
remain positive once exposure has occurred. They therefore
cannot be used to diagnose reinfection.

The venereal disease research laboratory test (VDRL) usually
becomes positive four to six weeks after an initial exposure, but will
return to negative again after approximately six months. Rising

VDRL titres are therefore used to monitor acute reinfections. False-positive VDRL results occur with several conditions, shown below. The levels in these disorders, however, are usually lower than 1:8.

- False-positive VDRL – infection (tuberculosis, malaria, viral hepatitis, EBV); mycoplasma; malignancy; chronic liver disease; connective tissue disorders; old age

Answer 11

(a) (i) Acute gastroenteritis   *(1 mark)*
     (ii) *Salmonella enteritidis*
          Campylobacter jejuni
          Enterotoxigenic *E. coli*   *(3 marks)*

(b) Foreign travel
     Contact with person exhibiting similar symptoms
     Both of the above are transmitted by faecal–oral
     crossinfection   *(2 marks)*

(c) Investigations:
         FBC, U&Es, glucose, LFTs
         Blood cultures
         Stool cultures
         Plain AXR
     Most cases are self-limiting and do not require
     any specific treatment
     More severe cases:
         Admit and isolate if possible
         Supportive treatment with analgesia, IV fluids
         and anti-emetics
         Antibiotic therapy may be appropriate when
         specific organisms are identified, eg salmonella
         Tracing of contacts and food source   *(4 marks)*

Comment

Gastroenteritis is a group of usually self-limiting disorders, characterised by diarrhoea and vomiting. They are spread through faecal–oral contamination, principally through contaminated water and foods. The onset of symptoms usually gives some indication of the causative organism, and it is therefore essential to try to obtain a clear history from the patient. For example, vomiting four to six hours after a meal is suggestive of toxin-producing *Staphylococcus aureus* infection, or *Bacillus cereus*. Pathogenicity is usually through one of two main mechanisms. *Vibrio cholerae*, enterotoxigenic *E. coli* and *Staphylococcus aureus* mediate their effects through toxin production. *Salmonella*, *Shigella*, rotavirus and *Campylobacter* cause mucosal damage with or without direct invasion. Most gastroenteritis requires only supportive treatment, ie. maintaining adequate hydration, anti-emetics and analgesia, if necessary. More serious cases, with a generalised systemic illness, require admission, isolation and treatment with antibiotics. Most organisms are sensitive to metronidazole or ciprofloxacin.

In patients where salmonella and *E. coli* species are isolated, contact tracing should be organised, particularly if the source is thought to be a cafe, restaurant, butcher or cooked meat suppliers, as these are notifiable illnesses in the UK.

Answer 12

(a) (i) Septic or septicaemic shock *(1 mark)*

(ii) Urinary tract infection secondary to the catheter
Intravenous cannula site infection
Postoperative chest infection *(3 marks)*

(b) FBC, U&Es, glucose
Clotting screen to include D-dimer and FDPs
Group and save
Blood cultures
Urine cultures
CXR
ECG
ABGs
Wound swab
Cannulae and catheter replaced and tips sent for culture; swab of cannulae sites *(3 marks)*

(c) Rapid assessment of the patient, trying to ascertain the cause of shock, ie sepsis site, myocardial infarction, gastrointestinal bleed, pulmonary embolism
Lie the patient flat if possible, with the foot of the bed raised
In this case:
    Re-site intravenous access
    Consider central venous line
    Start colloid infusion
    Broad spectrum antibiotics
    Oxygen via face mask
    Call senior colleague to assess   *(3 marks)*

Comment

Septicaemic shock in hospitalised patients is commonly associated with Gram-negative organisms from the urinary, gastrointestinal or biliary tract. Other causative organisms include *Streptococcus pneumoniae, Staphylococcus aureus* and *Staphylococcus epidermidis.* Prognosis is principally influenced by the patient's premorbid state and evidence of multi-organ involvement or failure. The presence of a normal or subnormal body temperature indicates a very poor prognosis. The condition continues to have significant associated mortality, particularly at the extremes of life. Various cytokines and leukotrienes are responsible for the inflammatory response to the infecting organisms which, in turn, cause shock and secondary multi-organ failure. It is hoped that by manipulation of these mediators the prognosis will eventually be improved. Please see www.survivingsepsis.com

Answer 13

(a) Amoebiasis with liver abscess
     Entamoeba histolytica   *(2 marks)*

(b) Liver abscess, which has caused hepatic enlargement, diaphragmatic irritation and referred shoulder pain
                                                          (2 marks)

(c) (i) FBC, LFTs and clotting screen
Stool culture – microscopy for ovum, cysts and parasites
Proctoscopy and rectal biopsy
Ultrasound scan of the liver
Ultrasound-guided aspiration of abscess – contents sent for MC+S *(3 marks)*

(ii) Treatment
Isolate the patient
Supportive treatment:
   Rehydration
   Nutritional support
   Analgesia for hepatic and shoulder pain
   Antibiotics, eg metronidazole
Followed by percutaneous aspiration of abscess under ultrasound or CT guidance *(3 marks)*

Comment

Amoebiasis may be divided into two forms. The non-invasive, asymptomatic form is characterised only by cyst excretion in the stool, and causes no associated mucosal pathology. The invasive form presents with an acute infective colitis, characterised by bloody diarrhoea and 'flask'-shaped ulcers within the mucosa. The colitis may be limited to a small area or present as a pancolitis. Haematogenous spread after mucosal invasion may cause hepatic abscess formation. This initially gives few systemic symptoms, but with enlargement progresses to cause swinging pyrexia, rigors and right upper quadrant pain. Diagnosis is confirmed by amoebic cysts in the stool, specific serological markers for amoebiasis and rectal or colonic biopsies. Hepatic involvement is demonstrated on ultrasound or CT scan, and is confirmed by cysts in the aspirated material. Treatment is principally medical with 75%–80% of cases responding to metronidazole or tinidazole. Diloxanide furoate is often given after the initial course of antibiotics to kill any remaining cysts within the colonic lumen. Slowly regressing abscesses are aspirated percutaneously under imaging, surgical drainage being rarely required. Complications of amoebiasis

CHAPTER 1 – ANSWERS

include colonic perforation, rupture of hepatic abscesses and extension of abscesses into the pleural and pericardial spaces, which require immediate drainage.

Answer 14

(a) (i) Parasitic worm infestation, eg strongyloides, filariasis, hookworm, roundworm   *(1 mark)*

(ii) Drug hypersensitivity and allergic disorders Asthma and polyarteritis nodosa   *(2 marks)*

(b) The respiratory symptoms are due to pulmonary eosinophilia   *(2 marks)*

(c) FBC with differential and blood film
U&Es, LFTs, glucose, calcium and phosphate, vitamin B12 and folate
Specific serological markers for parasitic worms
CXR
Stool culture
Duodenal aspirate via endoscopy   *(5 marks)*

Therapy is directed at the specific causative organism. Mebendazole, thiabendazole, albendazole and diethyl carbamazine are commonly used.

Comment

Parasitic worm infestations are common in tropical areas. They may present with malabsorption and weight loss and can produce a pulmonary eosinophilia, with asthma-like symptoms. Malabsorption may be confirmed on routine investigations by a raised MCV, low vitamin B12 and folate, low albumin and calcium. Infestation is confirmed by the presence of specific serological markers to the various organisms, isolation in stool cultures and duodenal aspirate. Pulmonary eosinophilia is the association of a peripheral eosinophilia with respiratory symptoms, such as dry cough and wheeze. The acute form is usually secondary to parasitic infection or drugs, eg NSAIDs or antibiotics. With continuing exposure this may develop into a chronic disorder. Other pulmonary conditions may present in this manner, eg asthma, polyarteritis nodosa and extrinsic allergic alveolitis. Other causes of eosinophilia include idiopathic hypereosinophilic syndrome, and haematological malignancies such as CML and lymphoma.

Answer 15

(a) (i) A fungus *(1 mark)*
(ii) Candidiasis – oropharyngeal and vaginal
Ringworm infection – *Trichophyton rubrum*
Athletes' foot – *Tinea pedis* *(2 marks)*

(b) CXR
Histoplasma antibody titres
Blood cultures
Sputum culture
In severe cases – bone marrow aspirate for MC+S
(3 marks)

(c) Amphotericin – nephrotoxic, hepatotoxic and cardiotoxic
Fluconazole – diarrhoea, Stevens–Johnson syndrome
Griseofulvin – peripheral neuropathy, photosensitivity, enzyme inducer
Itraconazole – peripheral neuropathy, cholestatic jaundice
Ketoconazole – hepatitis, gynaecomastia
Nystatin – rashes, diarrhoea
Terbinafine – diarrhoea, Stevens–Johnson syndrome
(4 marks)

Comment

Histoplasmosis is a fungal infection, which has two clinical forms, classical and African. Classical infection is caused by *Histoplasma capsulatum* which is found in the soil of endemic areas such as Australasia, South East Asia and the southern states of America. Its growth is particularly facilitated by the presence of bird excreta and bat guano, and therefore it is commonly found in caves where bats are nesting and around chicken farms. The infection may be divided into three main forms:

- Asymptomatic exposure and sensitisation – this accounts for 99% of cases
- Pulmonary disease
- Generalised systemic infection

Acute pulmonary disease occurs two to three weeks after an initial exposure, eg on a caving holiday. It presents with fever, malaise, and a non-productive cough, classically associated with erythema nodosum, and a flitting arthritis. Radiologically, the chest X-ray changes are often florid compared to the clinical condition of the patient, and there may be diffuse patchy shadowing and bilateral hilar lymphadenopathy. Usually only supportive treatment is necessary, but in more severe cases with associated hypoxia, intravenous antifungal agents are required.

Chronic pulmonary disease is principally seen in endemic areas, arising due to chronic exposure. It is particularly prevalent in male smokers with underlying airways disease. The resulting disease leads to pulmonary cavitation and fibrosis, and patients require antifungal therapy and, in more advanced cases, lobectomy.

Generalised systemic disease is principally seen at the extremes of life and in immunocompromised patients. It commonly affects the liver, spleen and bone marrow, but may also infiltrate the gut, central nervous system, and rarely the heart, causing endocarditis. The diagnosis is made by bone marrow and sputum culture and positive complement-fixing antibodies. Treatment is with intravenous itraconazole or amphotericin.

2

Metabolic Diseases

Answer 1

(a) Osteomalacia *(1 mark)*

(b) Low income hence poor diet, low in sources of vitamin D and calcium.
Phytate-containing flat bread flour may limit intestinal calcium absorption, increasing vitamin D requirement.
Cultural norms may limit exposure of skin to sunlight.
Efficiency of 25-hydroxylation of vitamin D may be reduced in pigmented (relative to White) skin.
Induction of hepatic enzymes by carbamazepine increases rate of vitamin D degradation. *(5 marks)*

(c) Obtain dietary history and provide advice if appropriate
Measure urine Ca^{2+} and serum U&E, LFT, bone profile, PTH and 25-hydroxy-vitamin D
Prescribe vitamin D supplements
Consider stopping carbamazepine *(4 marks)*

Comment

Rickets and osteomalacia are characterised by defective bone mineralisation, usually resulting from vitamin D deficiency. Rickets is the term used when defective bone mineralisation affects the growing skeleton, whereas osteomalacia is the term used when the same disease process affects adults. Childhood rickets causes deformity, with reduced growth velocity, bow-legs (genu varum), enlarged costo-chondral junctions, bossing of the skull and kyphosis being characteristic features. In contrast, adult-onset osteomalacia presents with proximal myopathy, bone pain and bone tenderness. Skeletal deformities are uncommon, with the exception of kyphosis. Typical investigation results include low serum and urine calcium, low serum 25-hydroxy-vitamin D and a compensatory increase in serum parathyroid hormone. Looser's zones may be seen on bone radiography, corresponding to areas of defective mineralisation.

Vitamin D deficiency arises from:

- Inadequate skin exposure to sunlight
- Inadequate diet
- Consumption of phytate-containing flour (eg in chapatti)
- Small bowel disease causing malabsorption
- Hepatic enzyme induction causing excessive degradation

Treatment for vitamin D deficiency is usually prescribed as ergocalciferol (calciferol or vitamin D_2) tablets with calcium supplementation. If malabsorption is suspected, or if adherence is a problem, an oily depot intramuscular injection is also available. In the presence of renal impairment or hypoparathyroidism, 1α-hydroxylated vitamin D_3 (alfacalcidol) or 1,25-dihydroxyvitamin D_3 (calcitriol) is useful.

Answer 2

(a) Kayser–Fleischer rings
Copper (Cu)   *(2 marks)*

(b) LFTs and clotting
Liver biopsy
Serum caeruloplasmin
Urinary copper   *(3 marks)*

(c) D-Penicillamine
Low copper diet
Consider liver transplant
Genetic counselling and family screening   *(5 marks)*

Comment

Wilson's disease (hepatolenticular degeneration) is an autosomal recessive disorder caused by mutations in the ATP7B gene on chromosome 13. The disorder arises due to defective metabolism of copper within the biliary tree, causing its deposition in various sites around the body. The principal sites affected are:

- Liver – the disease in its early stages produces mild hepatic dysfunction, but with progression produces cirrhosis with portal hypertension and oesophageal varices. Some patients present with chronic active hepatitis, which may conceal the underlying diagnosis
- Central nervous system – classically the disease produces an extrapyramidal movement disorder, with tremor, chorea and facial grimacing. Other presentations include dysarthria, dysphasia and parkinsonism. Frank psychiatric symptoms may also occur, but are usually in association with neurological symptoms and signs
- Eyes – the Kayser–Fleischer rings are due to copper deposition in Descemet's membrane of the cornea. They appear grey in dark eyes and brown in light-coloured eyes
- Kidneys – the disease is associated with an acquired Fanconi's syndrome, producing a type II (proximal) or a type IV (distal) renal tubular acidosis, depending on the site of predominant damage
- Cardiac – deposition of copper in the myocardium produces a cardiomyopathy and results in biventricular cardiac failure
- Skin and joints – the skin becomes a pigmented grey colour, whereas the joints may be hypermobile and premature osteoarthritis of the spine is common. Patients may develop a polyarthritis

Treatment is dependent on early recognition of the disease, and implementation of the chelating agent D-penicillamine. Liver transplant is potentially curative.

Answer 3

(a) Haemochromatosis
Accumulation of iron (Fe) in the body   *(3 marks)*

(b) FBC, glucose, LFTs, clotting
Serum Fe, ferritin, TIBC
USS of the liver and pancreas
Liver biopsy   *(4 marks)*

(c) (i)   Pancreatic infiltration leading to diabetes mellitus
(ii) Melanin deposition in the skin
(iii) Pyrophosphate arthropathy   *(3 marks)*

Comment

Primary haemochromatosis is an idiopathic disorder of iron metabolism, which is inherited in an autosomal recessive manner. The disorder leads to iron overload and deposition in various organs, including the liver, pancreas and the myocardium, causing cirrhosis, diabetes mellitus and a cardiomyopathy. The classical bronzed appearance is due to melanin deposition not iron. The diagnosis is confirmed by a raised serum iron[2] and a greatly increased saturation of the TIBC and serum ferritin. The liver disease is confirmed by biopsy. Treatment is aimed at lowering the iron level by regular venesection, which is performed at least once a week. Early detection and family screening dramatically improve the prognosis. Acquired iron overload, haemosiderosis, is most commonly seen in patients receiving repeated transfusions for chronic haemolytic diseases, particularly β-thalassaemia. The iron overload results from the transfusions and increased iron release. In these patients desferrioxamine may be used to chelate the excess iron.

Answer 4

(a) Familial hypercholesterolaemia (Fredrickson
hyperlipidaemia type IIa)
Autosomal dominant   *(2 marks)*

(b) Signs:
  Corneal arcus
  Tendon xanthoma
  Periorbital xanthoma
  Bedside tests:
  BM stix measurement
  Blood pressure
  Urinalysis for glycosuria   *(4 marks)*

(c) Address all other risk factors for atherosclerotic disease,
ie smoking, alcohol excess, obesity, hypertension,
diabetes mellitus
Dietician review – strict low-fat diet
Medical treatment – initially a member of the statin
group of lipid-lowering agents, eg simvastatin
Arrange sibling and family screening   *(4 marks)*

Comment

Familial hypercholesterolaemia is a common inherited disorder of
lipid metabolism which is particularly prevalent in the UK and
North America. It is caused by defective LDL catabolism, resulting
in an increase in LDL cholesterol. Patients' cholesterol levels are
usually in the range of 8–11 mmol/l. More uncommonly it is also
associated with an increase in VLDL, which causes an associated
hypertriglyceridaemia. Patients present with symptoms of
premature atherosclerotic disease, ie IHD, CVAs and peripheral
vascular disease. Hyperlipidaemia is classified by the
Fredrickson/WHO classification, as shown below:

Type	Lipoprotein increased	Lipid increased
I	Chylomicrons	Triglycerides (TGs)
IIa	LDL	Cholesterol
IIb	VLDL and LDL	TGs and cholesterol
III	Beta VLDL (IDL and chylomicron remnant)	TGs and cholesterol

In the mixed hyperlipidaemias, a fibrate is often added to a statin, to reduce the levels of triglycerides.

Answer 5

(a) The glycogen storage diseases   *(2 marks)*

(b) Autosomal recessive
Wilson's disease
Haemochromatosis
Sickle cell disease
Thalassaemia
Infantile polycystic kidney disease   *(4 marks)*

(c) Obtain a clear history from the parents, particularly a family history
Examination – short stature, obesity, hepatomegaly
Investigations – FBC, U&Es including bicarbonate, glucose, LFTs, clotting
Urinalysis
USS of liver and kidneys
Liver or renal biopsy for histological diagnosis
(4 marks)

Comment

The glycogen storage diseases are a rare group of disorders, caused by various enzyme defects in the metabolism or catabolism of glycogen. They therefore present with signs and symptoms of dysfunction of the two principal sites of glycogen utilisation, the liver and the skeletal muscle. They all share common features and present in the neonate or the first two years of life.

Those that mainly affect the liver, such as glucose-6-phosphatase deficiency (Von Gierke's disease), present with hepatomegaly, growth retardation and obesity. Von Gierke's disease classically presents with a bleeding tendency, as there is an acquired von Willebrand-like defect of the platelets, and attacks of hypoglycaemia and lactic acidosis. The diagnosis is confirmed by liver biopsy and specific histochemical staining. Treatment is aimed at maintaining normoglycaemia, which is achieved by overnight nasogastric glucose supplementation. This avoids the complications of hyperuricaemia and gout, hyperlipidaemia and acidosis, which in turn promotes normal growth and a much improved prognosis. Without such treatment the patient develops increasing hepatic and renal dysfunction, leading to premature death. These patients are at risk of developing hepatocellular carcinoma. Disorders principally affecting the musculature, eg Pompe's disease, present with a generalised defect of cardiac and skeletal muscle, with associated hepatic abnormalities. They carry a poor prognosis and the patients do not survive beyond the age of one or two years. There is no specific treatment.

Answer 6

(a) Sweating, palpitations and pyrexia
Motor weakness
Mania, depression, hallucination   (*2 marks*)

(b) Drugs, eg benzodiazepines
Acute infection
Prolonged fasting
Oestrogen and progesterone, eg pregnancy and
the oral contraceptive pill   (*3 marks*)

(c)   Acute:
      Analgesia (opiates)
      Remove the precipitating factor
      Propranolol for symptoms of sympathetic
      overactivity
      Haematin therapy
      Ensure adequate carbohydrate intake if signs of
      motor neuropathy – consider ITU for assisted
      ventilation
    Prevention: education of the patient with
    regard to possible precipitating factors   *(5 marks)*

Comment

The porphyrias are a group of disorders that arise due to various enzyme defects in the haem synthesis pathway. They are divided into acute and non-acute porphyrias. The acute porphyrias, acute intermittent, variegate and hereditary coproporphyria, are characterised by acute attacks, triggered by environmental agents. Acute intermittent porphyria is the commonest, and is inherited in an autosomal dominant manner. It is five times more common in women, principally due to oestrogen hormones in the oral contraceptive pill and during pregnancy. Biochemically they are characterised by an excess of urinary porphobilinogen and delta aminolaevulinic acid. Clinically the patient may present with severe abdominal pain and vomiting, which may resemble an acute abdomen. The other acute porphyrias may also present with a photosensitive rash, due to excess porphyrin production. Drugs are a common precipitating factor in the acute presentations. Drugs that may cause an acute attack include: tricyclic antidepressants and MAOIs; barbiturates and benzodiazepines; antibiotics, sulphonamides and cephalosporins; diuretics and sulphonylureas. The non-acute porphyrias are *porphyria cutanea tarda*, congenital porphyria and erythropoietic protoporphyria. *Porphyria cutanea tarda* is characterised by a photosensitive bullous rash, which produces scarring on healing. It may be precipitated by alcohol, and is associated with mild iron overload, which leads to chronic liver disease. Treatment includes regular venesection and chloroquine, which increases urinary excretion of uroporphyrin. Congenital porphyria is a rare autosomal recessive disorder producing a severe photosensitive bullous rash, which causes disfiguring scarring. Erythropoietic protoporphyria is an autosomal dominant disorder, which produces pain and discoloration of the skin on exposure to sunlight, associated with chronic liver disease. Treatment with β-carotene improves the skin condition.

Answer 7

(a) Tay-Sach's disease
Inflammatory bowel disease   (*2 marks*)

(b) (i) Sphingolipidoses
Autosomal recessive   (*2 marks*)
(ii) FBC
Clotting screen LFTs
USS of the liver and spleen   (*3 marks*)

(c) There is a relatively good prognosis in the absence of neurological symptoms
Therapeutic management:
Enzyme replacement
Correction of the anaemia
Consider splenectomy
Bisphosphonates   (*3 marks*)

Comment

The sphingolipidoses are a group of disorders caused by the defective catabolism of sphingolipid, leading to an accumulation of various intermediary degradation products. The accumulation of these molecules occurs within the lysosomes of specific tissues, such as the central nervous system, the liver, spleen, lungs and the bone marrow, which, in turn, produces varying patterns of clinical presentation. In the diseases affecting the central nervous system, there is often retinal involvement, with the characteristic 'cherry red spot' at the macula. Gaucher's disease is due to glucocerebrocidase deficiency, and has three clinical variants, all of which present with hepatosplenomegaly and the pathognomonic

Gaucher cells in the bone marrow. The commonest variant does not involve the nervous system and presents in childhood with hepatomegaly, massive splenomegaly, and symptoms secondary to splenic enlargement and bone marrow infiltration. Treatment with enzyme replacement, using macrophage-targeted glucocerebrocidase and bisphosphonates, which improve the bony complications, have both improved overall prognosis. Patients with severe marrow dysfunction require bone marrow transplant. The variants that affect the central nervous system present with seizures, cognitive impairment and focal neurological deficit. The more malignant of the two is associated with pulmonary infiltration, leading to recurrent sepsis and death in the first year of life.

Answer 8

(a) Autosomal recessive *(1 mark)*

(b) High arched palate, lens dislocation, genu valgum, scoliosis
Pectus carinatum is a 'pigeon chest' *(4 marks)*

(c) Presenting complications are a left calf DVT, with associated pulmonary embolism
Therapeutic management:
IV access
Anticoagulate – initially with intravenous heparin, then with warfarin (aiming for an INR of 2–3)
Analgesia *(5 marks)*

Comment

Homocystinuria is an aminoacidopathy arising due to an enzyme deficiency in the methionine/cysteine pathway. The defective gene is on chromosome 21. It usually presents in late childhood or early adulthood, with low IQ, lens dislocation, skeletal abnormalities and thromboembolic disease. Visual problems are common, arising due to the lens dislocation, glaucoma and retinal detachment. The patients share several features of Marfan's syndrome, but are distinguished by their low IQ. Classically they have a thrombotic tendency, and commonly present with DVT and pulmonary emboli. There is also a predisposition to premature atheromatous disease. Treatment is based on reducing the levels of methionine and homocysteine by the use of oral pyridoxine. In those unresponsive to this treatment, a methionine-free, low-protein diet is used.

Answer 9

(a) Metabolic acidosis
Liver failure
Circulatory failure
Renal failure   *(3 marks)*

(b) Correct extracellular fluid and electrolyte deficits via Na^+ and water depletion by IV isotonic NaCl solution
Isotonic $NaHCO_3$ solution to replace impaired renal regeneration of bicarbonate; this also has a positive inotropic effect on the heart
Dialysis may be required if treatment induces Na overload   *(4 marks)*

(c) Methanol, ethanol
Ethylene glycol
Paraldehyde
Metformin
Paracetamol   *(3 marks)*

Comment

The correction of acidosis by $NaHCO_3$ infusion may improve cardiac function and peripheral circulation, alleviate hyperventilation and correct hyperkalaemia. However, rapid alkalinisation in an effort to lower H^+ may reduce cerebral blood flow and reduce oxygenation of the blood. $NaHCO_3$ as an alkalinising agent may also cause Na overload and, paradoxically, may acutely increase intracellular acidosis by $\uparrow p(CO_2)$. Liver and renal function must be closely monitored.

Answer 10

(a) Lactic acidosis due to increased production of lactic
acid in severe exercise leading to lactic acid
accumulation in tissues, producing a
metabolic acidosis
Dehydration and salt depletion due to loss of water
and salt in sweat during severe exercise, particularly
in hot weather   *(4 marks)*

(b) Administer oxygen by face mask to convert lactic acid
to pyruvic acid and reduce air hunger
IV infusion of isotonic dextrose saline to maintain
circulatory volume and to provide substrate for
aerobic metabolism
Provide warmth with blankets to prevent heat loss
from chilling   *(2 marks)*

(c) Dehydration and Na loss – assessed by serum U&E and
corrected by appropriate IV fluid therapy
Metabolic acidosis assessed by ABG would correct itself
as accumulated lactic acid is progressively oxidized to
pyruvic acid and increased respiratory effort washes
out the CO_2 *(4 marks)*

Comment

Lactic acidosis occurs in otherwise healthy individuals as a result
of shock leading to circulatory failure, or severe exercise resulting
in anaerobic metabolism in muscle tissue, both of which result in
lactic acid accumulation. The use of $NaHCO_3$ infusion to correct
the acidosis is hazardous: although it may improve cardiac output
and peripheral circulation and correct hyperkalaemia, it shifts the
O_2 dissociation curve to the left and reduces cerebral perfusion,
thereby precipitating cerebral hypoxia.

3

ANSWERS

Neurology

Answer 1

(a) Right hemisphere stroke leading to left hemiparesis
Right middle cerebral artery   *(2 marks)*

(b)

	UMN	LMN
Bulk	Normal	Normal or wasted
Tone	Increased hypertonia	Decreased hypotonia
Reflexes	Hyperreflexia ± clonus	Hyporeflexia
Plantars	Extensor (upgoing)	Flexor (downgoing)

(2 marks)

(c) Investigations:
   FBC, U&Es, glucose, ESR, lipid profile
   ECG
   CXR
   CT head scan
   Consider Doppler USS of the carotids ± angiography
                                        (3 marks)

Therapeutic management will be based on the cause of
the stroke, which is confirmed by CT scan
In thromboembolic stroke:
   Add aspirin 300 mg od
   Consider anticoagulation with warfarin – indications
   include atrial fibrillation, thrombus in the left
   ventricle and an enlarged left atrium

All stroke patients should be considered for expert multidisciplinary rehabilitation involving physiotherapy, occupational therapy, speech therapy, and liaison between district services and social workers   *(3 marks)*

Comment

Cerebrovascular disease remains one of the three primary causes of death in the Western world, with an annual incidence of approximately 2:1000 of the population. A stroke is defined as 'an acute episode of focal or global loss of cerebral function, lasting for more than 24 hours, or as the principal cause of death'. There are three main causes:

- Cerebral infarction – this accounts for 80% of all strokes
- Intracerebral haemorrhage – 10%
- Subarachnoid haemorrhage – 10%

The risk factors for stroke include:

- Hypertension – this is the main aetiological risk factor and its control has a greater effect than in cardiovascular disease
- Increasing age
- Smoking
- Alcohol abuse
- Cardiac disease – ischaemic, valvular disease, paroxysmal tachyarrhythmia, eg atrial fibrillation
- Past history of, or known TIAs or stroke
- Diabetes mellitus
- Hyperlipidaemia
- Peripheral vascular disease
- The oral contraceptive pill – increases risk two- to threefold
- Hypercoagulable states – hyperosmolar coma
- Malignancy
- Systemic vasculitides – SLE
- Hypotensive episodes – myocardial infarction, during anaesthesia

Answer 2

(a) Sub-arachnoid haemorrhage *(1 mark)*

(b) Migraine
Stress headache
Meningitis
Space-occupying lesion
Sagittal sinus thrombosis (particularly if she is on the
oral contraceptive pill) *(3 marks)*

(c) Investigations:
FBC, U&Es, glucose
CXR
CT head scan
Consider lumbar puncture
Therapeutic management:
Nurse in a quiet room if possible
IV access and fluids
Analgesia (opiates if necessary)
Nimodipine
Neurosurgical opinion *(6 marks)*

Comment

Sub-arachnoid haemorrhage is responsible for 10% of all strokes.
The majority of patients bleed after rupture of a saccular
intracranial aneurysm or from an arteriovenous malformation.
Clinically the patient presents with a severe headache, which starts
abruptly and is often described as the worst headache they have
ever experienced. It may be associated with neck stiffness,
meningism and occasionally seizures. Consciousness may be
impaired, and the patient may present in coma with larger bleeds.
Diagnosis is usually confirmed with CT head scan, which will
show blood in the ventricles and sub-arachnoid space. (Blood
appears as a white collection on an unenhanced scan.) A lumbar
puncture may be required if the scan is unhelpful and, if
confirmatory, will show blood in all three CSF samples. A sample
taken 24 hours or more after the initial symptoms may appear

yellow in colour, termed xanthochromia. Fifty per cent of patients will die within one month of their initial episode. Neurosurgical intervention should always be considered when the patient is neurologically intact and consciousness is spared. Radiological embolisation of arteriovenous malformations now offers a less invasive method of treatment. The calcium-channel blocker nimodipine is recommended for secondary prophylaxis, as it stops vasospasm causing secondary bleeds. It may be given orally or intravenously depending on the patient's level of consciousness.

Answer 3

(a) Horner's syndrome
Loss of the sympathetic nerve supply to the eye
(2 marks)

(b) (i) An apical malignant tumour in the right lung
(Pancoast's tumour)   *(1 mark)*
(ii) Brainstem stroke
Syringomyelia
Accidental or surgical trauma to the neck
(3 marks)

(c) A right third nerve palsy causes the full ptosis, with the action of the unopposed superior oblique and lateral rectus muscles causing the eye to turn down and out. Loss of the parasympathetic nerve supply causes the fixed, dilated pupil.
Causes:
Diabetes mellitus
Mononeuritis multiplex
Midbrain stroke   *(4 marks)*

Comment

The Horner's syndrome consists of enophthalmos, the globe of the eye being sunken in the orbit, pupillary constriction, partial ptosis and anhidrosis, or loss of sweating on the affected side of the face (this is dependent on whether the interruption of the nerve supply is above or below the cervical sympathetic ganglion). The syndrome arises due to an interruption in the sympathetic nerve supply to the eye. This may arise anywhere along its course from the midbrain, down through the brainstem and cervical cord, as it emerges from the spine at Tl, and then as it passes up through the neck. Common lesions are:

- Brainstem – stroke, tumours, syringobulbia
- Cervical cord – tumour, syringomyelia
- T1 lesion – Pancoast's tumour, benign apical lung disease, eg TB or abscess
- In the neck – operative or accidental cervical trauma.

In apical lung disease, the brachial plexus may also be involved leading to pain, paraesthesia and loss of sensation along the ulnar border of the forearm and the medial (ulnar) two fingers, as well as wasting of the intrinsic muscles of the hand. Third nerve palsies may occur in isolation or with loss of the accompanying parasympathetic nerve supply. If the parasympathetic supply is unaffected this is termed 'papillary sparing', which arises principally due to a vascular event.

Answer 4

   (a) (i) Left facial (seventh) nerve palsy   *(1 mark)*

        (ii) Lower motor neurone lesions cause a total hemifacial palsy, whereas upper motor neurone lesions have sparing of the forehead and the upper eyelid   *(2 marks)*

   (b) Idiopathic
Parotid infiltration
Pontine tumours and stroke
Mononeuritis multiplex   *(4 marks)*

   (c) Bell's palsy
In early presentations high-dose steroids are advocated
Most will resolve spontaneously   *(3 marks)*

Comment

Facial nerve palsy is a common cranial nerve lesion, most often presenting as part of a stroke. The nerve innervates the muscles of facial expression, and supplies taste sensation to the anterior two-thirds of the tongue. The facial nucleus lies within the pons and receives bilateral motor cortex supply. Thus lesions that are supranuclear cause an upper motor neurone palsy and have sparing of the superior aspects of the face due to contralateral nerve supply. Common causes of a facial palsy are:

- Upper motor neurone – pontine stroke, tumours, cerebral cortex and internal capsule stroke
- Lower motor neurone – idiopathic (Bell's palsy), cerebellopontine angle tumours, Ramsey Hunt syndrome (this is caused by a herpes zoster infection), basal skull fracture, parotid infiltration (eg sarcoid, lymphoma, amyloid), iatrogenic injury during facial and parotid surgery, mononeuritis multiplex (eg diabetes mellitus, systemic vasculitides)

Answer 5

(a) (i) Peripheral sensory neuropathy *(1 mark)*
   (ii) Malignancy
     Alcohol abuse *(2 marks)*

(b) Light touch, proprioception and vibration – dorsal columns
  Pinprick (pain) and temperature – spinothalamic tract *(3 marks)*

(c) Stroke (CVA)
  Mononeuritis multiplex
  Autonomic neuropathy
  Cranial nerve palsies
  Argyll Robertson pupil *(4 marks)*

Comment

Peripheral sensory neuropathy is a common sequela of poorly controlled diabetes mellitus. It is thought to occur as a result of both microvascular disease and disturbance of axonal metabolism, causing secondary damage to nerve conduction. Other common causes of neuropathy are:

- Sensory neuropathy
  Idiopathic (50%)
  Metabolic – diabetes mellitus, B12 deficiency, uraemia, hypothyroidism
  Drugs – isoniazid, phenytoin, chloramphenicol
  Alcohol associated – thiamine (vitamin B1) deficiency
  Malignancy – as part of a paraneoplastic phenomenon.
- Motor neuropathy
  Heavy metal toxicity – lead, mercury
  Drugs – gold, amphotericin
  Motor neurone disease
  Malignancy – paraneoplastic phenomenon
  Guillain–Barré syndrome

Answer 6

(a) Benign and malignant tumours
Obstructing hydrocephalus
Benign intracranial hypertension *(3 marks)*

(b) CT or MRI scan of the brain (with contrast)
CXR
FBC with blood film and differential
If appropriate – HIV test with pretest counselling *(3 marks)*

(c) Neurosurgery:
    Drainage of abscess
    Biopsy of mass
    Excision of accessible masses
  Radiotherapy:
    Curative, palliative or adjuvant
  Chemotherapy:
    Monotherapy or adjuvant
  Medical:
    Antibiotics for abscesses   *(4 marks)*

Comment

This woman gives a history suggestive of raised intracranial pressure, with headache, nausea and vomiting, visual disturbance and seizures, which are common presenting symptoms. Focal neurological deficit may present as third and sixth cranial nerve palsies with an ipsilateral hemiparesis, and are known as 'false localising signs'. They are due to increasing intracranial pressure stretching the nerves at the base of the skull. Causes of raised intracranial pressure include:

- Infection (meningitis, abscess), benign tumours (meningioma, neurofibroma), malignant tumours (primary – astrocytoma, glioma, neuroblastoma, lymphoma; secondary – cervical, breast, lung)

Obstructing hydrocephalus may be secondary to:

- Tumours of the posterior fossa
- Subarachnoid haemorrhage
- Tuberculous meningitis
- Colloid cyst of the third ventricle

Benign intracranial hypertension is an idiopathic disorder, commonly seen in young women. It is thought to be related to obesity and the oral contraceptive pill. Patients present with severe headaches for which the only abnormality found is raised intracranial pressure. Treatment is based on stopping the pill, weight reduction and diuretics. Normal pressure hydrocephalus is a syndrome seen principally in the elderly, which presents with a classical triad of worsening confusion, urinary incontinence and dyspraxia. The diagnosis is confirmed by CT head scan, which shows dilatation of the ventricles without evidence of cerebral atrophy. Lumbar puncture will confirm normal manometry. Although single manometry readings are normal, these patients often have periods of raised intracranial pressure and may benefit from insertion of a ventriculoperitoneal shunt.

Answer 7

(a) Epilepsy – probably absence seizure   *(1 mark)*

(b) FBC, U&Es, glucose, calcium and magnesium
     CXR
     MRI head scan
     EEG
     Lumbar puncture   *(5 marks)*

(c) Sodium valproate – ataxia, jaundice
     Carbamazepine – gynaecomastia, GI upset
     Phenytoin – seizures, peripheral neuropathy, gingival,
     hyperplasia, folate deficiency
     Phenobarbitone – megaloblastic anaemia, confusion,
     sedation
     Lamotrigine – rashes, fever
     Vigabatrin – drowsiness, confusion
     Gabapentin – drowsiness, ataxia   *(4 marks)*

Comment

Epilepsy is a common neurological disorder, with an annual incidence of 80:100 000 cases in the UK. It is defined as two or more non-febrile seizures. Epilepsy is classified into three groups, which are subdivided by the characteristics of the seizures:

- **Partial seizures** are caused by the activation of a localised, definable group of neurones, sited within one cerebral hemisphere. They are subdivided into: **simple partial seizures** – these are characterised by the site of the abnormal activity, eg pure motor, sensory or psychic phenomena; they are not associated with loss of consciousness; **complex partial seizures** – these have the symptoms of simple seizures, but are associated with an impairment of consciousness; **secondary generalised seizures** – these begin with features of simple or complex seizures, which then become generalised with tonic–clonic episodes. The initial partial element may be so short-lived that it may be only evident on the EEG

- **Generalised seizures** arise due to symmetrical abnormal neuronal activation in the cerebral hemispheres. They are subdivided as **absence seizures** and **myoclonic seizures**. **Absence seizures** are subdivided into typical and atypical. Typical absence seizures are characterised by their EEG discharge of 3 Hz 'spike and waves', and were formerly known as *petit mal* seizures. Both are associated with impaired consciousness, with typical seizures often associated with complex patterns of movement and behaviour. **Myoclonic seizures** are sub-divided into tonic–clonic (formerly known as *grand mal* seizures), tonic and clonic seizures. They are associated with impairment of consciousness. Classically tonic–clonic seizures are associated with biting of the tongue and incontinence of urine.

Answer 8

(a) Motor neurone disease
Progressive bulbar palsy   *(3 marks)*

(b) EMG
Myelogram
Muscle biopsy
MRI of the cervical spine and brainstem
Lumbar puncture   *(3 marks)*

(c) Once other diagnoses have been excluded:
    An experienced physician should discuss the
    prognosis, and counsel the patient and family
    Speech therapist to improve articulation and
    swallowing
    Physiotherapy and occupational therapy
    Nutrition support and dietary advice, may require
    gastrostomy feeding
    Computer-assisted communication for speech
    failure or severe dysarthria
    Terminal care – community support, eg Macmillan
    nurses, hospice care   *(4 marks)*

Comment

Motor neurone disease is an idiopathic, progressive neurological
disorder, characterised by a mixture of upper and lower motor
neurone signs. There are never associated sensory or cerebellar
signs and the ocular movements are preserved. It is a diagnosis of
exclusion as there are no definitive tests for the disorder and the
diagnosis can therefore only be inferred clinically and by negative
investigations for the main differential diagnoses. MRI of the
cervical spine and brainstem, with or without myelography, is the
principal investigation, as this will exclude the main differential,
cervical spondylosis with associated radiculomyelopathy. Motor
neurone disease is one of the main causes of a progressive bulbar
palsy, ie palsies of the ninth to twelfth cranial nerves, which lie
within the medulla or bulb of the brainstem. Patients present with
'nasal' speech and dysarthria, and dysphagia to both solids and
liquids. The tongue is wasted and flaccid and there is weakness of
palatal movement. Other causes include syringobulbia,
Guillain–Barré syndrome and poliomyelitis. Motor neurone
disease carries a poor prognosis and there is no specific treatment,
but riluzole (Rilutek®) slows progression of the disease. Palliation
is the main aim of therapy, requiring a multidisciplinary approach.
The prognosis is mainly dependent on the involvement of the
bulbar muscles. In cases where the initial symptoms are spinal,
15% survive to five years; if there are associated bulbar symptoms
this falls to approximately 5%.

Answer 9

(a) Myasthenia gravis
Autoimmune disease – autoantibodies (IgG) directed
against the postsynaptic acetylcholine (ACh)
receptor   (3 marks)

(b) Tensilon (edrophonium) test
Autoantibody screen including the IgG directed against
the ACh receptor   (2 marks)

(c) Oral anticholinesterases, eg pyridostigmine
Immunosuppressants – steroids and azathioprine
Thymectomy – in patients under 40 years old
Plasma exchange – in short-term control
Atropine – cholinergic crisis   (5 marks)

Comment

Myasthenia gravis is an autoimmune disease caused by an
autoantibody IgG, directed against the postsynaptic acetylcholine
receptor. It is associated with several other autoimmune disorders
including thyrotoxicosis and myxoedema, pernicious anaemia,
rheumatoid arthritis and SLE. It occurs at most ages, but has a peak
incidence at 30. As with most autoimmune disorders it is more
common in women. The thymus gland is often abnormal in these
patients, especially in those under 40 years old. Some 60%–70%
have thymic hyperplasia and 10% develop a thymoma. This group
of patients commonly has an additional autoantibody directed
against striated muscle. A thymectomy is recommended in this
group, especially in the under 40s. The diagnosis is usually
confirmed by a Tensilon test. An intravenous injection of an
anticholinesterase (edrophonium) is given, which produces an
instant improvement. If the initial injection fails to do so, a further
larger bolus can be given. Lambert–Eaton syndrome is a
malignancy-associated myasthenic syndrome, most often
occurring as a result of a small cell tumour of the lung. Unlike the
primary disorder, the IgG is directed against the presynaptic
calcium channels, and so it does not respond to anticholinesterases.

Treatment is directed at the underlying tumour and increasing the action potential duration and the amount of neurotransmitter released using the drug 3,4-diaminopyridine.

Answer 10

(a) Parkinson's disease
   Dopamine *(2 marks)*

(b) Arteriosclerotic or vascular Parkinson's syndrome
   Drug-induced parkinsonism
   Progressive supranuclear palsy
   (Steele–Richardson–Olszewski syndrome) *(2 marks)*

(c) L-dopa – nausea, confusion, postural hypotension
   Selegiline – confusion, hypotension
   Pergolide and other ergotamine derivatives –
   hallucination, recently shown to cause cardiac
   valvular fibrosis
   Apomorphine – hallucination, nausea
   Bromocriptine – confusion *(6 marks)*

Comment

Parkinson's disease is a common neurological disorder, particularly in the elderly, where its prevalence is 1:200. It classically presents with an insidious onset of bradykinesia, rigidity and tremor, associated with postural and gait problems. This combination leads to increasing difficulties with mobility and falls. Pathologically it is characterised by an idiopathic loss of dopaminergic cells within the substantia nigra, and the presence of eosinophilic inclusions, known as Lewy bodies. In parkinsonism, the extra-pyramidal, akinetic rigidity symptoms arise in relation to other diffuse brain disease, such as vascular dementia, Alzheimer's disease, Lewy body dementia, and Creutzfeldt–Jakob disease. Parkinsonism may also arise secondary to various toxic insults to the brain, eg anoxia, carbon monoxide poisoning, and drugs such as antipsychotics and antiemetics. Parkinson's disease is treated initially with a combination of L-dopa and a peripheral dopa decarboxylase inhibitor, which will improve symptoms but do not influence the progression of the disease. As the disorder progresses, other agents may be employed. These include the dopamine agonists pergolide, lisuride and bromocriptine, and the MAOI type B, selegiline. In difficult cases, where there is a poor response to medication, or in advanced disease, a continuous subcutaneous infusion of apomorphine may be used. Surgical intervention may also be tried in these cases, using stereotactic thalamotomy and thalamic stimulation. The implantation of fetal dopaminergic tissue remains controversial.

Answer 11

(a) (i) X-linked recessive   *(1 mark)*
(ii) Becker's muscular dystrophy
Lesch–Nyhan syndrome
Haemophilia A
Red–green colour blindness   *(2 marks)*

(b) CK
Muscle biopsy
EMG   *(3 marks)*

(c) Drugs, eg steroids
Infection – poliomyelitis
Endocrine – Cushing's syndrome, hypothyroidism
Toxins – alcohol   *(4 marks)*

Comment

Duchenne's muscular dystrophy is classically an X-linked recessive disorder, although one-third of cases arise due to spontaneous mutation. The responsible gene defect is located in the Xp21 region of the X chromosome. The condition presents in early childhood with wasting of the proximal limb musculature, and associated weakness. The child walks with a 'waddling' gait and classically cannot 'walk' their hands up their legs to a standing position (Gower's sign). The proximal wasting is often associated with enlargement of the calves, termed pseudohypertrophy. The disorder is progressive and the child is often confined to a wheelchair by the age of 10, with death occurring by the age of 20 due to cardiac and respiratory muscle involvement. Becker's muscular dystrophy is a more benign disorder, which presents usually in the second to third decade of life and progresses slowly with the patient usually confined to a wheelchair by the age of 40–50.

Answer 12

(a) Multiple sclerosis
     Plaques of demyelination within the central nervous
     system   *(2 marks)*

(b) CSF for oligoclonal bands
     MRI of the cervical spine and brainstem to
     demonstrate plaques of demyelination
     Visual evoked responses (VER) show delayed
     conduction between the retina and the occipital
     cortex   *(3 marks)*

(c) Education about the disease and prognosis for patient
     and family
     In relapses – high-dose IV methylprednisolone
     Symptom relief and help for:
          Incontinence
          Spasticity
          Immobility
          Sexual dysfunction
     Social support for patient and family   *(5 marks)*

Comment

Multiple sclerosis is an idiopathic disorder, causing demyelination within the central nervous system. It presents between the ages of 20 and 40 years. It is a disease principally of northern Europeans, and the immigrant populations of South Africa and Australasia that descended from them. The disease is thought to be due to an abnormal immune response to environmental agents, such as viruses, as a direct result or as a consequence of abnormal gene sequencing. Viral agents implicated in this immune reaction include measles, mumps, rubella and EBV. The disease is divided clinically into a chronic progressive disorder and a rapid relapsing/remitting one. Prognosis is at present uninfluenced by any treatments, and therapy is principally aimed at palliation of the complications and delay of relapses with immunosuppressants. Relapses are shortened in duration by high-dose intravenous steroids. Beta interferon is the most promising of the conventional therapies, and work is also continuing into the use of monoclonal antibody therapy directed against the abnormal immunological responses.

Answer 13

(a) (i)   This woman has spinal metastases from her colonic carcinoma   *(1 mark)*
     (ii) Extrinsic and intrinsic spinal cord lesions
           Demyelination
           Trauma   *(2 marks)*

(b) T10 is approximately the level of the umbilicus
     X-rays of the thoracic and lumbar spine
     Radioisotope bone scan
     MRI ± myelography of the spinal cord   *(4 marks)*

(c) Management:
         Neurosurgical decompression of the cord
         Local radiotherapy to bony metastases
     Palliation of symptoms:
         Urinary catheter for incontinence
         Laxatives for constipation
         Analgesia
     Multidisciplinary palliative care team   *(3 marks)*

Comment

A spastic paraparesis may present insidiously, worsening over several months, or as an acute event. In all cases it is essential to define whether a sensory level is present, and to what extent bladder and anal sphincter control are affected. Common causes of a spastic paraparesis are:

- Extrinsic cord compression – this is principally due to infiltration or collapse of the vertebral bodies. Common causes include: metastases, eg bronchus, breast, prostate, thyroid and colon; myeloma; Paget's disease of the bone; Pott's disease of the spine (tuberculosis); spondylolysthesis
- Other causes of external compression are tumours, eg neurofibroma, meningioma and abscesses
- Intrinsic cord lesions (tumours, eg ependymoma, glioma, teratoma; demyelination; syringomyelia; metabolic, eg vitamin B12 deficiency; vascular, eg anterior spinal artery occlusion)

Answer 14

(a) (i) Guillain–Barré syndrome *(1 mark)*
   (ii) Paraneoplastic syndrome
      Infective, eg HIV
      Hereditary sensorimotor neuropathy *(2 marks)*

(b) Hypotonia with loss of power
   Diminished or absent patella and ankle reflexes
   Flexor plantar responses
   Fasciculation may occur *(3 marks)*

(c) Management:
     Usually supportive treatment only, ie nutrition, fluids, bed rest
     Treat any reversible cause, eg *Mycoplasma pneumoniae*
     Monitor respiratory function with regular spirometry
     May require assisted ventilation
     If prolonged will require nutritional support
     If severe, consider plasma exchange and IV human immunoglobulin *(4 marks)*

Comment

Guillain–Barré syndrome is a postinfective polyneuropathy, which has recently been closely linked to *Campylobacter jejuni* and HIV infection, particularly in its more malignant form. Other implicated organisms include EBV, CMV, enterovirus and *Mycoplasma pneumoniae*. In 40% of cases there is no identifiable preceding cause. The disorder commonly presents one to three weeks after the onset of the infection, with distal motor and sensory symptoms and signs. In 20% of cases the symptoms ascend to involve the respiratory and facial muscles, causing acute respiratory failure and the need for assisted ventilation. In these severe cases plasma exchange and human immunoglobulin are often required. High-dose steroids are commonly given but do not influence the outcome. Other causes of a sensorimotor neuropathy include:

- Hereditary sensorimotor neuropathies (eg Charcot–Marie–Tooth disease)
- Malignancy (paraneoplastic syndrome)
- Infection (HIV, Lymes' disease, diphtheria)
- Amyloid

Answer 15

(a)   Autosomal dominant
1:2 chance   *(2 marks)*

(b)   Chorea – continuous, irregular movements which may be explosive in nature, and flit from one part of the body to another
Other causes:
  Sydenham's chorea
  Chorea gravidarum
  Drugs, eg neuroleptics
  Thyrotoxicosis   *(4 marks)*

(c)   Genetic counselling and screening of patient and family
Exclude any treatable causes
Palliation of symptoms – phenothiazines and tetrabenazine are given for the chorea; antipsychotics
Social support for family and patient
Consider nursing home care if family are unable to cope with patient at home   *(4 marks)*

Comment

Huntington's chorea is a progressive neurological disorder, characterised by a relentlessly progressive dementia and choreiform movements. There are adult and childhood forms, the early onset being between 10 and 20 years and the adult form between 30 and 50 years. The abnormal gene locus has been isolated to the short arm of chromosome 4, which has allowed genetic screening of family members, including the foetus in utero. Pathologically the disorder is characterised by loss of GABA and ACh within the corpus striatum and ACE and metenkephalin within the substantia nigra. The loss of these neurotransmitters leads to a relative excess of dopaminergic activity, which is thought to be responsible for the choreiform movements. Other causes of chorea include:

- Sydenham's chorea (this is associated with rheumatic fever but may occur in association with other disorders; chorea gravidarum is regarded as a variant of this condition and occurs in pregnancy and with users of the oral contraceptive pill)
- Drugs (neuroleptics, anticonvulsants)
- Toxins (alcohol)
- Benign hereditary chorea
- Endocrine disorders (thyrotoxicosis, hypoparathyroidism)
- Metabolic (hypernatraemia)
- Intra-cranial haemorrhage and thromboembolic strokes
- Polycythaemia rubra vera

Answer 16

(a) Ataxic, wide-based gait
Past pointing
Intention tremor
Dysdiadochokinesis
Cerebellar (staccato) speech
Horizontal nystagmus   (2 marks)

(b) Chronic alcohol abuse
Phenytoin toxicity   (2 marks)

(c) Investigations:
      FBC with MCV
      LFTs including gamma GT
      Phenytoin level
   Medications:
      Diazepam or chlormethiazole for
      withdrawal symptoms
      Multivitamins and thiamine   *(6 marks)*

Comment

Cerebellar lesions may present with ipsilateral or bilateral signs, depending on the cause. They are characterised by problems of movement control and co-ordination. Dysmetria is the inability to control the force, direction and distance of a movement, whilst dysdiadochokinesia is the inability to perform rapid alternating movements. Patients with cerebellar lesions classically have staccato speech and coarse, horizontal nystagmus; they may also have hypotonia and diminished reflexes. Common causes of cerebellar lesions include:

- Cerebellar infarction or haemorrhage
- Cerebellar abscess
- Demyelination
- Toxins (eg alcohol, lead, carbon monoxide)
- Drugs (eg anticonvulsants)
- Inherited disorders (eg Friedreich's ataxia, ataxia–telangiectasia)
- Anatomical abnormalities (eg Arnold–Chiari malformation, Dandy–Walker syndrome)
- Malignancy (primary and secondary tumours; a paraneoplastic syndrome)

Endocrinology

Answer 1

(a) (i) Hypoglycaemia
Diabetic ketoacidosis
(ii) Hyperosmolar non-ketotic (HONK) state
Lactic acidosis (complication of metformin
treatment)   *(2 marks)*

(b) Urine ketones – for evidence of ketoacidosis
Arterial blood gases – for severity of acidosis and to
confirm metabolic source
Urea and electrolytes – to check for hyperkalaemia and
renal impairment
Plasma glucose (laboratory assay) – to confirm
capillary blood meter reading
Electrocardiogram – for evidence of hyperkalaemia
(2 marks)

(c) Two venous cannulae, preferably in large veins
ECG monitoring
Intravenous fluids: 0.9% saline 1 l over the first hour
Insulin: Soluble insulin 12 units IV bolus
followed by an IV infusion of
6 units/hour (fixed rate, not sliding
scale)
Potassium: 20 or 40 mmol in second litre of IV
fluid
Speed of subsequent fluid replacement guided by
clinical examination, blood pressure and urine output.
Probably 4–6 l over the first 24 hours.
Type of fluid, and amount of potassium replacement,
guided by repeated U&E measurements. Consider

0.45% saline if serum sodium elevated.
Urinary catheterisation once treatment started.
Reduce insulin infusion rate to 3 units/hour once
plasma glucose ≤ 12 mmol/l and continue at this rate
until ketones gone. Use glucose infusion to prevent
hypoglycaemia if necessary.
Restart subcutaneous insulin at least one hour
before stopping insulin infusion   *(6 marks)*

Comments

Diabetic ketoacidosis is a life-threatening emergency. It is most
commonly associated with type I diabetes mellitus, either as a result
of inadequate insulin administration (eg during intercurrent
illness) or as the presenting feature of newly diagnosed diabetes.
More rarely it may occur with type II diabetes mellitus, particularly
in patients of sub-Saharan African ethnic origin. It is essential that
people with type I diabetes mellitus learn that they become insulin
resistant during intercurrent illness and, hence, that their insulin
requirements increase. Ketoacidosis is most likely to develop when
a patient's appetite is reduced as a result of, for instance, food
poisoning. Insulin treatment should always continue in this
situation, and doses may need to increase despite reduced food
intake. For this reason, people with type I diabetes mellitus should
carry with them a set of 'sick day rules', agreed with their diabetes
service, which provide instructions on what to do during illness.

Answer 2

(a)   Abuse of androgenic (anabolic) steroids   *(1 mark)*

(b)   Alcohol abuse
      Cannabis use
      Haemochromatosis
      Drug-induced hyperprolactinaemia
      Klinefelter's syndrome
      Pituitary tumours
      Hypothalamic tumours
      Kallman's syndrome
      SRY translocation   *(5 marks)*

(c) Obtain adequate history, especially social circumstances and drug use

Examine, including the external genitalia

Fasting plasma glucose

FBC

Serum prolactin, LH, FSH, testosterone, iron studies and LFTs

Urinary steroid profile, urine toxicology for exogenous androgenic steroids and cannabis   *(4 marks)*

Comment

This patient's history strongly suggests use of androgenic steroids. Spermatogenesis requires both testosterone and stimulation of the Sertoli cells by FSH. Oligozoospermia has occurred because exogenous androgens have suppressed pituitary gonadotrophin (FSH and LH) release. It is common for patients who abuse androgenic steroids to deny that they are doing so, even if they are not involved in competitive sport.

Causes of male infertility are categorised as primary (ie testicular failure) or secondary (ie failure of pituitary gonadotrophin release). Secondary hypogonadism is also known by endocrinologists as hypogonadotrophic hypogonadism, mainly because it sounds impressive and difficult to understand.

Causes of primary hypogonadism:

- Alcohol
- Cannabis
- Haemochromatosis – causes both primary and secondary hypogonadism as a result of iron deposition in the testes and anterior pituitary, respectively. Other pituitary cell types, eg corticotroph, thyrotroph, are unaffected. Other effects of haemochromatosis include diabetes mellitus and hepatic cirrhosis
- Klinefelter's syndrome (karyotype 47, XXY) – semen analysis usually reveals azoospermia but severe oligozoospermia may occur in a minority of individuals with mosaic 47, XXY/46, XY karyotypes, and a very small number of spontaneous pregnancies have been reported

CHAPTER 4 – ANSWERS

- SRY translocation – karyotype 46, XX with a short length of paternal Y chromosome, including the testis determining factor (SRY) gene translocated onto one of the X chromosomes. Always azoospermic

Causes of secondary hypogonadism:

- Haemochromatosis – causes primary and secondary hypogonadism – see above
- Exogenous androgens – the same mechanism, using oestrogens rather than androgens, provides the basis for the female combined oral contraceptive pill
- Drug-induced hyperprolactinaemia – dopamine receptor antagonists, eg antipsychotics, some anti-emetics
- Hyperprolactinaemia from secretion by a lactotroph pituitary adenoma (prolactinoma)
- Other tumours, inflammation or trauma affecting the pituitary gland or hypothalamus
- Kallman's syndrome – anosmia (absent sense of smell) and failure of the hypothalamus to secrete luteinising hormone releasing hormone (LHRH, also known as gonadotrophin releasing hormone type I). The pituitary gland is normal but is not stimulated to release gonadotrophins
- Idiopathic hypogonadotrophic hypogonadism – similar to Kallman's syndrome but sense of smell unaffected

Answer 3

(a) Polycystic ovary syndrome (PCOS)
Late-onset 21–hydroxylase deficiency *(2 marks)*

(b) Gonadotrophins (early follicular phase if feasible)
Oestradiol
Prolactin
Sex hormone binding globulin
Testosterone, DHEAS, androstenedione
17–hydroxyprogesterone
Ultrasound scan of the ovaries *(4 marks)*

   (c) Weight-reducing, low-carbohydrate diet
        Subsequent treatment dependent on principal problem
        and reproductive intentions:

- Hirsutism: eflornithine cream
- Hirsutism and acne: oral contraceptive pill (OCP) ± cyproterone acetate
- Irregular menses/infertility: metformin clomiphene
- Potential additions: spironolactone (especially if hypertensive) or finasteride for androgenic symptoms resistant to above measures. NB Any anti-androgen to be prescribed only in the presence of robust contraceptive measures, eg OCP, depot progesterone, progesterone implant, progesterone-releasing intra-uterine system or conventional copper coil
- Discuss association between PCOS and the risk of developing type 2 diabetes mellitus. Emphasise importance of diet and exercise   *(4 marks)*

Comment

Diagnosis of polycystic ovary syndrome (PCOS) requires, firstly, exclusion of other conditions that may mimic its features, eg adrenal or ovarian carcinoma or late-onset 21–hydroxylase deficiency, and, secondly, the presence of two out of three of:

- menstrual cycle disturbance (ranging from irregular cycles to severe, anovulatory oligomenorrhoea causing infertility)
- clinical (ie acne and/or hirsutism) and biochemical evidence of hyperandrogenaemia
- polycystic ovaries (seen on cross-sectional imaging, eg ultrasound, or at laparoscopy)

The severity of symptoms varies widely but it is inappropriate to diagnose PCOS in an entirely asymptomatic woman when an incidental finding of polycystic ovaries is made during investigation for an unrelated complaint.

Hyperinsulinaemia is central to the pathological basis of PCOS. It sensitises the ovaries to the effects of luteinising hormone, leading to increased androgen synthesis and to the arrest of normal follicular development. Weight loss and metformin, which improve insulin sensitivity, are thus useful for every feature of PCOS. Further treatments are symptom-directed. Acne and hirsutism respond to an oral contraceptive pill, to which cyproterone acetate, an anti-androgen, is frequently added. Hirsutism may also be improved by eflornithine cream. Ovulation and fertility may require clomiphene, recombinant follicle-stimulating hormone or in vitro fertilisation.

Answer 4

   (a) (i) Primary hypothyroidism   *(1 mark)*

        (ii) Autoimmune thyroiditis:
                Hashimoto's thyroiditis
                Atrophic thyroiditis
            Other thyroiditis:
                Subacute (De Quervain's) thyroiditis
                Riedel's thyroiditis
            Drug-induced:
                Thionamide drugs, eg carbimazole, propylthiouracil
                Amiodarone
                Lithium
            Other iatrogenic hypothyroidism:
                Thyroidectomy
                Radioiodine (131I), eg for Graves' disease
                External beam radiotherapy to the neck
            Iodine deficiency
            Congenital hypothyroidism:
                Thyroid dysgenesis
                Dyshormonogenesis   *(2 marks)*

(b) Replacement therapy with oral thyroxine for life, with a starting dose of 50 mcg per day. Titrate every two to three weeks, usually to a dose of 100 to 150 µg per day, aiming to restore serum TSH to the lower half of the normal range. Starting dose and rate of titration are more cautious in the elderly and in patients with ischaemic heart disease where a dose of 25 mcg is commonly used   *(3 marks)*

(c) Myxoedematous coma is a medical emergency. Triiodothyronine and thyroxine are administered IV until clinical improvement allows substitution with oral thyroxine. Mechanical ventilation, circulatory support and reversal of hypothermia are commonly necessary

(4 marks)

Comment

Autoimmune thyroiditis is the commonest cause of primary hypothyroidism in the UK. In Hashimoto's disease, lymphocytic infiltration causes goitre formation, whereas atrophic thyroiditis results in fibrosis and reduction in size of the thyroid gland. The two processes may overlap and both are associated with high titres of antithyroglobulin and antithyroid peroxidase antibodies. TSH-receptor blocking antibodies may also be present, particularly in atrophic thyroiditis.

Subacute (De Quervain's) thyroiditis is typified by tender thyroid enlargement and transient thyrotoxicosis early in the illness. Hypothyroidism follows but often resolves spontaneously after a few months.

The mortality in severe hypothyroidism in the elderly is significant and may manifest as confusion dementia or coma. Hypothermia, cardiac failure, hypoventilation, hypocalcaemia and hyponatraemia may all be present, and the patient should be managed in an intensive therapy unit.

Answer 5

(a) Thyrotoxicosis secondary to Graves' disease. TSH receptor antibodies stimulate follicular cells in the thyroid gland, causing uncontrolled production of thyroid hormones *(3 marks)*

(b) Diffuse goitre with bruit
Signs of thyrotoxicosis:
    Sinus tachycardia/atrial fibrillation
    Sweating/warm peripheries
    Lid lag and lid retraction
    Proximal myopathy
Signs of Graves' ophthalmopathy:
    Swollen eyelids
    Chemosis
    Proptosis
    Ophthalmoplegia
    Diplopia
    Corneal involvement
    Sight loss
Pretibial myxoedema
Thyroid acropachy *(3 marks)*

(c)

Treatment:	Complications:
Antithyroid (thionamide) drugs, eg carbimazole, propylthiouracil	Rashes Agranulocytosis Relapse after stopping therapy
Sub-total or near-total thyroidectomy	Hypothyroidism Recurrent thyrotoxicosis Hypoparathyroidism Recurrent laryngeal nerve injury
Radioiodine therapy	Hypothyroidism Exacerbation of eye disease

(4 marks)

Comment

Graves' disease, the commonest cause of thyrotoxicosis, results from stimulation of thyroid follicular cell TSH receptors by autoantibodies. The thyroid gland becomes diffusely enlarged and hypervascular, often resulting in the presence of a bruit. Graves' ophthalmopathy affects 30%–40% of sufferers but is eight to ten times more common, and usually more severe, in smokers. Pretibial myxoedema and thyroid acropachy are rare but characteristic features. Together these 3 features (achropachy, ophthalmopathy and pretibial myxoedema) are known as 'Graves' triad'.

Thionamide drugs are the usual first-line treatment in the UK. The chance of long-term remission after a standard course of treatment is slightly less than 50%. If the disease recurs, long-term remission is very unlikely to be achieved by a second course, so definitive treatment is usually offered. Radioiodine is effective, safe and inexpensive. Hypothyroidism often occurs but is much easier to manage than fluctuating thyrotoxicosis. Sub-total or near-total thyroidectomy is an alternative to radioiodine and is more likely to be considered for young patients and those with large goitres and/or severe eye disease.

Answer 6

(a) (i) Lactotroph pituitary microadenoma
(microprolactinoma) *(1 mark)*
(ii) Pregnancy *(1 mark)*

(b) Antipsychotics, eg chlorpromazine, haloperidol, risperidone
Anti-emetics, eg metoclopramide, domperidone
Antidepressants, eg amitriptyline, fluoxetine, venlafaxine
Oestrogens
Methyldopa *(4 marks)*

(c) Exclude pregnancy (human chorionic gonadotrophin assay in serum or urine)
Check for assay interference by macroprolactin
MRI pituitary
Dopamine agonist therapy with cabergoline or bromocriptine, aiming to suppress serum prolactin into normal range   *(4 marks)*

Comment

Causes of hyperprolactinaemia include:
Pregnancy
Lactation
Drugs – see above
Polycystic ovary syndrome
Renal failure (because of reduced/absent renal clearance of prolactin)
Primary hypothyroidism (because of stimulation of lactotroph cells by TRH)
Prolactin-secreting pituitary tumours (lactotroph pituitary adenomas)
Non-prolactin-secreting pituitary or hypothalamic masses, eg non-functioning pituitary adenomas, Craniopharyngioma, lymphocytic hypophysitis, pituitary sarcoidosis
Assay interference by macroprolactin

Prolactin is secreted by the anterior pituitary gland under inhibitory control by hypothalamic dopamine.
Hyperprolactinaemia in the presence of a pituitary tumour thus results either from secretion of prolactin by a tumour composed of lactotroph cells (a prolactinoma), or because compression of the pituitary gland and stalk interferes with the normal flow of dopamine from the hypothalamus to the anterior pituitary. This distinction is very important in clinical practice, since lactotroph adenomas shrink and may resolve entirely with dopamine agonist treatment, whereas other tumours generally require surgery and/or radiotherapy.

An important step, when hyperprolactinaemia is first identified in a patient, is to check for the presence of macroprolactin in the serum

sample. Macroprolactin (not to be confused with
macroprolactinoma, which is another term for a lactotroph
pituitary adenoma of greater than 1 cm diameter) is a non-immune
complex of prolactin with IgG. It is biologically inactive but it
interferes in prolactin assays, causing artefactually elevated results.

Answer 7

(a) (i) Acromegaly caused by a somatotroph
(growth hormone-secreting) pituitary
adenoma   *(2 marks)*
   (ii) Oral glucose tolerance test showing failure
to suppress serum growth hormone   *(2 marks)*

(b) Sweating
Macroglossia
Prognathism
Interdental separation
Hypertension
Carpal tunnel syndrome
Obstructive sleep apnoea syndrome
Kyphosis
Headache
Bitemporal hemianopia
Hypopituitarism   *(3 marks)*

(c) Hypophysectomy (usually transsphenoidal but
transfrontal for tumours with large suprasellar
extension)
Pituitary radiotherapy
Somatostatin analogue, eg octreotide, lanreotide
Dopamine agonist, eg cabergoline, bromocriptine
Growth hormone receptor antagonist, eg pegvisomant
                                                    (3 marks)

Comment

Acromegaly results from excessive secretion of growth hormone,
usually from a somatotroph pituitary adenoma. If the tumour
develops prior to fusion of the epiphyses, gigantism results. Excess

growth hormone and insulin-like growth factor-I (IGF-I) cause soft tissue expansion, giving rise to the characteristic enlargement of the extremities and coarsening of facial features. Metabolic effects are also prominent, especially insulin resistance and hypertension, and the risk of cardiovascular and respiratory disease is substantially elevated. The majority of patients with acromegaly present with pituitary macroadenomas, ie tumours greater than 1 cm in diameter that typically expand outside the pituitary fossa. Such expansion may cause headaches, hyperprolactinaemia, hypopituitarism, cranial nerve palsies and compression of the optic chiasm resulting in visual field defects.

Answer 8

(a)   (i)   Cushing's syndrome is defined as the clinical state caused by prolonged inappropriate elevation of circulating glucocorticoids

(ii) • Exogenous glucocorticoid exposure:
   – Iatrogenic
   – Illegal 'herbal remedies'
  • Endogenous glucocorticoid exposure:
   – ACTH-dependent:
    ○ corticotroph pituitary adenoma (Cushing's disease)
    ○ Ectopic ACTH syndrome
   – ACTH-independent:
    ○ Adrenal adenoma
    ○ Adrenal carcinoma
    ○ Macronodular adrenal hyperplasia

(3 marks)

(b) Round ('moon') face
Facial plethora
Interscapular fat pad ('buffalo hump')
Purplish striae
Hirsutism or hair loss
Menstrual disturbance
Loss of libido
Lethargy
Depression
Psychosis
Osteopenia
Impaired glucose tolerance   (3 marks)

(c) (i) Urinary free cortisol
Overnight dexamethasone suppression test
(1 mg at 23:00 hours)
48-hour low-dose dexamethasone suppression test
(0.5 mg six-hourly)
Sleeping midnight serum cortisol
(ii) Plasma ACTH level at 09:00 hours
Serum potassium and bicarbonate
High-dose dexamethasone suppression test
Corticotrophin-releasing hormone (CRH) test
Bilateral inferior petrosal sinus sampling (for
plasma ACTH levels)   (4 marks)

Comment

The commonest cause of Cushing's syndrome is the use of exogenous glucocorticoids, usually prescribed for the management of chronic inflammatory diseases but, not infrequently, also found in supposedly 'herbal' remedies. Endogenous Cushing's syndrome, on the other hand, is a rare condition. The majority of cases are ACTH-dependent. Cushing's disease, defined as Cushing's syndrome caused by an ACTH-secreting corticotroph pituitary adenoma, accounts for 80% of these. Ectopic sources of ACTH secretion include small cell lung carcinoma and bronchial carcinoid tumours. Radiological techniques, particularly pituitary MRI, thoracic CT scanning and either CT scanning or MRI of the adrenals, are vital in discovering the cause of confirmed Cushing's syndrome. Nonetheless, they should not be employed until the diagnosis has been proved biochemically, since false positives occur frequently and may cause considerable confusion.

Answer 9

(a) (i) Addison's disease
(ii) Infectious adrenalitis:
Tuberculosis
Fungal infections, eg histoplasmosis
Autoimmune adrenalitis
Primary or secondary neoplasia
Bilateral adrenal haemorrhage:
In severe sepsis (Waterhouse-Friderichsen syndrome)
Trauma
Extensive burns
Coagulopathy
Inherited steroidogenic pathway enzyme defects:
21-hydroxylase deficiency
11β-hydroxylase deficiency   (*3 marks*)

(b) Nausea
Vomiting
Anorexia
Hypotension with postural drop
Abdominal pain
Diarrhoea
Vitiligo   (*3 marks*)

(c) (i) Hyponatraemia
Hyperkalaemia
(ii) Simultaneous 09:00 hours serum cortisol and plasma ACTH.
Short synacthen test (tetracosactrin 250 µg IV or IM with serum cortisol measurements at baseline, 30 min and 60 min. Normal result is serum cortisol > 550 nmol/l at 30 min)   (*4 marks*)

Comment

Autoimmune destruction is the commonest cause of Addison's disease in the UK, although tuberculosis is more common worldwide. Autoimmune Addison's disease frequently occurs as part of a polyglandular autoimmune syndrome, the commonest associations being hypo- or hyperthyroidism, type I diabetes mellitus and testicular or ovarian failure. Since the entire adrenal cortex is destroyed, production of both cortisol and aldosterone is lost. Addison's disease is thus treated with oral hydrocortisone (cortisol) and fludrocortisone (a synthetic mineralocorticoid). Cortisol requirements increase in times of stress, so the oral dose of hydrocortisone should be doubled during intercurrent illnesses. In severe illness, or when nausea, vomiting or torrential diarrhoea prevent absorption of oral hydrocortisone, the intravenous or intramuscular routes should be used instead. In acute adrenal crisis, intravenous fluids are also necessary to restore circulating volume. Patients with Addison's disease should be advised to carry at all times a steroid card and a bracelet or neck chain stating their diagnosis and treatment.

Answer 10

(a) Renin-independent, excessive aldosterone secretion arising either from an adrenal adenoma (Conn's syndrome) or from bilateral adrenal hyperplasia. Aldosterone excess leads to urinary potassium and hydrogen ion loss, along with hypertension. *(4 marks)*

(b) Hypokalaemia
Metabolic alkalosis
Urinary potassium inappropriately high
Low plasma renin
Elevated plasma aldosterone *(3 marks)*

(c) An adenoma may be surgically removed.
Bilateral adrenal hyperplasia is treated with the aldosterone antagonist spironolactone (100–400 mg/day), or with amiloride (10–40 mg/day) *(3 marks)*

Comment

Aldosterone is the mineralocorticoid hormone secreted by the zona glomerulosa of the adrenal cortex. In health, its secretion is regulated by the renin–angiotensin system. Primary hyperaldosteronism is the term given to autonomous (ie renin independent), excessive aldosterone secretion. It accounts for approximately 5% of cases of treatment-resistant hypertension, of which one-third result from a solitary adrenal adenoma (Conn's syndrome) and two-thirds result from bilateral adrenal hyperplasia.

Conn's syndrome is one of the few surgically curable causes of hypertension. However, the biochemical abnormalities of primary hyperaldosteronism are often subtle and may be masked by standard hypertension treatment. Furthermore, there are usually no other clues to the underlying diagnosis except for resistance to standard therapy. A low threshold for further investigation is therefore justified when hypokalaemia is observed in a hypertensive patient.

Further investigations commence with a urine potassium concentration. If this is high, implying urinary potassium wasting, plasma renin and aldosterone should be assayed. Various electrolyte disturbances and drugs alter renin and aldosterone levels (see table). Other investigations include a therapeutic trial of spironolactone; postural studies; oral salt loading; the intravenous saline load test; fludrocortisone suppression testing; adrenal vein sampling, and adrenal imaging, including CT scanning, MRI and scintigraphy. If a surgical cure is not possible, hypertension secondary to primary hyperaldosteronism may respond to spironolactone or amiloride. Amiloride is usually preferred for men because of the incidence of gynaecomastia with high-dose spironolactone.

Table: Effects of electrolyte disturbances and antihypertensives on renin and aldosterone levels

Drug or condition	Effect
Beta-blockers	↓ Renin
Salt depletion	↑ Renin and aldosterone
Loop and thiazide diuretics	↑ Renin and aldosterone
Mineralocorticoid receptor antagonists	↑ Renin and aldosterone
Hypokalaemia	↓ Aldosterone
Calcium channel blockers	↓ Aldosterone
Angiotensin-converting enzyme (ACE) inhibitors	↓ Aldosterone
Angiotensin II receptor antagonists	↓ Aldosterone
Alpha-adrenoceptor antagonists	Negligible

Answer 11

(a) Desmopressin acts on V2 receptors in the renal collecting ducts to promote water reabsorption and, hence, to render urine more concentrated. Urine concentration should rise to ≥750 mOsmol/kg

(3 marks)

(b) (i) Cranial (or hypothalamic, or central) diabetes insipidus

(ii) Desmopressin intranasal spray
Desmopressin tablets
Desmopressin injection (usually only in hospital)
Conservative management   *(4 marks)*

(c)   **Traumatic**, eg head injury, neurosurgery
Neoplastic, eg craniopharyngioma, germinoma,
metastatic deposits in hypothalamus or pituitary
Inflammatory, eg sarcoidosis or tuberculosis affecting
the pituitary, lymphocytic hypophysitis, autoimmune
Vascular, eg Sheehan's syndrome (pituitary infarction)
Pregnancy   *(3 marks)*

Comment

Diabetes insipidus arises from an inability to concentrate urine
adequately. It is classified as cranial when vasopressin release is
impaired, and nephrogenic when the kidneys fail to respond to
vasopressin. In addition to the causes listed in the answer to part
(c) above, cranial diabetes insipidus may occur in infancy as a
feature of inherited and developmental abnormalities. Causes of
nephrogenic diabetes insipidus are listed below.

Mild cranial diabetes insipidus (urine volume up to 4 l per
24 hours) is often managed conservatively. Larger urine volumes
require treatment with desmopressin, an analogue of vasopressin.
Since unregulated desmopressin treatment may result in life-
threatening hyponatraemia, patients should allow themselves to
become polyuric and thirsty at least once a week. The management
of cranial diabetes insipidus in patients without an intact sense of
thirst is fraught with difficulty.

Causes of nephrogenic diabetes insipidus include:

• Inherited defects of vasopressin receptor or aquaporin genes
• Chronic renal disease, eg polycystic kidney disease
• Drug-induced, eg lithium toxicity (not necessarily in overdose)
• Osmotic, eg hypercalcaemia.

Answer 12

(a) (i) Calcium in the blood exists in both ionised (physiologically active) and albumin-bound (inactive) forms. The extent of binding varies with the albumin level. Serum calcium is therefore corrected by convention to the serum albumin level

(ii) Parathyroid adenoma causing primary hyperparathyroidism   *(2 marks)*

(b) Malignancy with lytic bone lesions, eg multiple myeloma, metastases of breast or bronchial carcinoma
Non-metastatic ('humoral') paraneoplastic hypercalcaemia
Granulomatous disease, eg sarcoidosis, tuberculosis
Vitamin D toxicity
Paget's disease with immobilisation
Milk-alkali syndrome
Thyrotoxicosis
Addison's disease   *(3 marks)*

(c) Stop the thiazide diuretic (because it inhibits urinary calcium excretion). Rehydrate with 4–6 l of intravenous normal saline in the first 24 hours, with added potassium if necessary. Continue intravenous fluids until the patient is rehydrated and serum calcium is below 3 mmol/l. Once the patient is rehydrated, consider expediting parathyroidectomy. Bisphosphonates (eg pamidronate infusion), corticosteroids and calcitonin are often used in the management of acute severe hypercalcaemia but are rarely indicated for primary hyperparathyroidism. Calcimimetic therapy (eg cinacalcet) may be an alternative to surgery   *(5 marks)*

Comment

Primary hyperparathyroidism is a common condition, usually presenting in middle age and resulting from a solitary parathyroid adenoma. Parathyroid carcinoma is rare but causes more severe hypercalcaemia. Primary hyperparathyroidism is also a feature of several inherited conditions, including the multiple endocrine neoplasia (MEN) syndromes. Patients with MEN type I frequently develop multiple-gland hyperplasia, rather than a solitary adenoma.

The effects of long-standing hyperparathyroidism include renal stone formation, osteitis fibrosa cystica and muscle weakness. However, such severe manifestations are very infrequent and primary hyperparathyroidism is often an almost asymptomatic illness. Non-specific symptoms of hypercalcaemia include fatigue, weakness, depression and poor concentration. Osteoporosis and vascular calcification are also promoted by continuously elevated parathyroid hormone levels.

Parathyroidectomy is the only cure for primary hyperparathyroidism and is a safe procedure in experienced hands. Nonetheless, a significant proportion of patients with mild disease opt for conservative management. Calcimimetic drugs, which are already licensed for use in secondary hyperparathyroidism and parathyroid carcinoma, may become an accepted part of treatment for these patients as well.

Answer 13

(a) Phaeochromocytoma
Acute anxiety state
Thyrotoxicosis
Paroxysmal atrial tachycardia
Carcinoid syndrome
Autonomic epilepsy   *(2 marks)*

(b) (i) Phaeochromocytoma
(ii) Establish α-adrenoceptor blockade, followed by β-blockade
CT and/or MRI scan adrenal glands
[131I]metaiodobenzylguanidine (mIBG) and/or octreotide scintigraphy
Selective venous sampling for noradrenaline levels if imaging fails to localise the lesion   *(5 marks)*

(c) Surgical excision
Combined α- and β-adrenoceptor blockade with oral phenoxybenzamine (20–40 mg/day) initially, then propranolol (120–140 mg/day). Intravenous phenoxybenzamine added for 2–3 days prior to surgery   *(3 marks)*

Comment

Catecholamine-secreting tumours arising in the adrenal medulla are termed phaeochromocytomas, whereas extra-adrenal tumours are known as paragangliomas. Most are benign, although the risk of malignancy is higher with paragangliomas. Both tumour types may occur in familial cancer syndromes, including von Hippel–Lindau syndrome and multiple endocrine neoplasia type IIa and IIb. Phaeochromocytomas and paragangliomas present in a similar fashion. Hypertension may be continuous or intermittent but the symptoms of catecholamine excess typically occur in paroxysms, and are sometimes interpreted by the patient as panic attacks. Hypertensive crisis may occur, precipitating myocardial infarction, acute renal failure, stroke and/or sudden death. Such crises may occur spontaneously or as a result of medical interventions, including abdominal examination and radiographic contrast injection. Patients under investigation for possible phaeochromocytoma or paraganglioma should therefore be treated with adrenergic blocking agents. α-Adrenoceptor blockade should always be commenced before β-blockade, because unopposed α-adrenoceptor stimulation may itself precipitate potentially fatal hypertensive crisis.

Answer 14

(a) Type I diabetes mellitus
Diabetic ketoacidosis
Type II diabetes mellitus *(3 marks)*

(b) Urgent urinalysis for ketones
Urgent laboratory assay of plasma glucose
Elicit family history of diabetes mellitus
Examine for features of insulin resistance, eg acanthosis nigricans
Examine for long-term complications of diabetes mellitus, eg retinopathy
Glutamic acid decarboxylase (GAD) and islet cell autoantibody assays *(3 marks)*

(c) Assessment of ketones is first priority. If suggests diabetic ketoacidosis, arrange emergency admission to hospital. Whether or not ketones are present, the patient has suffered dramatic weight loss and has marked hyperglycaemia. She therefore needs insulin treatment acutely.
Long-term treatment depends on diagnosis: if type I diabetes mellitus, continue subcutaneous insulin.
If type II, she will probably benefit from switch to metformin. Metformin will reduce insulin resistance and may improve her symptoms of polycystic ovary syndrome *(4 marks)*

Comment

In addition to causing long-term complications, hyperglycaemia has osmotic effects, which often constitute the presenting features of diabetes mellitus. The renal tubular reabsorption threshold for glucose is overwhelmed, resulting in loss of glucose in the urine and, hence, an osmotic diuresis. This leads to polyuria (large urine volume) and polydipsia (excessive thirst). In combination with a catabolic state induced by insulinopaenia, these symptoms also cause weight loss and lethargy. Hyperglycaemia also results in alteration to the refractive properties of the cornea and lens, causing blurred vision.

The ideal treatment regimens for diabetes mellitus vary according to the type. It is thus important to establish the type at, or soon after, the time of diagnosis. As a worst-case scenario, misdiagnosis of a patient with type I disease (autoimmune destruction of pancreatic islet β-cells, leading to total loss of endogenous insulin production) may lead to diabetic ketoacidosis and death. On the other hand, misdiagnosis of a patient with type II disease (insulin resistance with gradual loss of β-cell secretory function) may lead to unnecessary weight gain on insulin treatment. Other groups of patients with relatively uncommon genetic forms of diabetes (eg maturity-onset diabetes of the young – MODY – see www.diabetesgenes.org) may require either no treatment or may be more effectively treated with sulphonylurea tablets than with insulin.

Answer 15

(a) Background: microaneurysms, retinal haemorrhages, exudates
Preproliferative: venous beading or looping, more extensive haemorrhages, intraretinal microvascular abnormalities
Proliferative: new vessels, preretinal or vitreous haemorrhage, preretinal fibrosis or tractional retinal detachment
Maculopathy is classified in parallel, describing changes occurring within one optic disc diameter of the fovea

(3 marks)

(b) Polyuria
Erectile dysfunction
Frequent infections
Lethargy
Weight loss
Neuropathic burning pain *(3 marks)*

(c) Biguanides: metformin
     Thiazolidinediones: pioglitazone, rosiglitazone
     Alpha-glucosidase
        inhibitors: acarbose
     Sulphonylureas: eg gliclazide, tolbutamide
     Meglitinides: nateglinide, repaglinide
     Insulins: eg insulin detemir, insulin
                                       glargine
     Incretin mimetics: eg exenatide   *(4 marks)*

Comment

Type II diabetes mellitus is characterised initially by insulin
resistance, with a gradual decline in pancreatic β-cell function
occurring subsequently. It is strongly associated with obesity,
hypertension and dyslipidaemia. In contrast to type I diabetes
mellitus, the onset of type II disease is rarely dramatic. Affected
individuals often ignore osmotic symptoms of hyperglycaemia
(polyuria, polydipsia, blurred vision, lethargy) for several years
before coming to medical attention. As a result, newly diagnosed
patients may present with complications of long-standing
diabetes. These are classified as:

• Microvascular:
  – eye disease: diabetic retinopathy, rubeosis iridis
  – nephropathy
  – neuropathy: stocking distribution sensory neuropathy (leading
                to foot ulceration or Charcot's foot deformity)
                autonomic neuropathy
                mononeuritis multiplex
                diabetic amyotrophy
• Macrovascular:
  – coronary artery disease (angina, myocardial infarction)
  – cerebral vascular disease (stroke)
  – peripheral vascular disease (lower limb ischaemia, gangrene)

The risk of complications in all forms of diabetes mellitus may be
minimised by maintaining a conventionally healthy lifestyle, by
adequately controlling blood pressure (ideally using lower target

values than are suitable for the non-diabetic population), by maintaining excellent glycaemic control and by using lipid-lowering therapies, such as statins. Certain antihypertensive medications, eg angiotensin-converting enzyme inhibitors, are especially effective at preventing diabetic nephropathy and other complications.

5

Respiratory Medicine

Answer 1

(a) Reduced expansion on side of effusion
Deviation of trachea away from the effusion
Reduced tactile vocal fremitus
Stony dull percussion note
Reduced or absent breath sounds
Reduced vocal resonance
Whispering pectoriloquy sometimes occurs in consolidated/atelectatic lung just above the upper border of the effusion   *(3 marks)*

(b) (i) Simple parapneumonic effusion
Empyema
(ii) Aspiration pneumonia   *(3 marks)*

(c) Investigations:
FBC, clotting screen, arterial blood gases (on room air)
Venous blood cultures, sputum sample for microscopy, culture and sensitivity
Chest radiograph
Diagnostic aspirate of effusion – send for microbiology (Gram stain, AAFB stain, culture and sensitivity), protein, lactate dehydrogenase, pH and cytology. However, if it looks and smells like pus, only microbiology is necessary

Treatment:
   Analgesia
   Oxygen therapy as per arterial blood gases
   Antibiotics: IV cefuroxime + IV metronidazole until
   sensitivities available
   If effusion turbid, purulent or foul-smelling, or
   pH < 7.2, or LDH > 1000 IU/l, insert intercostal
   drain and refer to respiratory physician   *(4 marks)*

Comment

Empyema is a collection of pus in the pleural cavity. It is a
life-threatening condition that arises after disseminated
bacteraemia, trauma or, more usually, as a complication of
pneumonia. Empyema occurs most commonly in the setting of
hospital-acquired pneumonia, severe community-acquired
pneumonia and aspiration pneumonia. It must be differentiated
from simple parapneumonic effusion, which occurs in up to 50%
of all cases of pneumonia and which, in contrast to empyema, may
be treated conservatively.

The diagnosis is based on examination of a pleural aspirate. This
may usually be obtained in the Emergency Department or on the
ward using a 21G (green) needle and a 50-ml syringe. If the
effusion is small or loculated, it may be necessary for it to be
aspirated under ultrasound guidance. If the fluid is purulent and
foul smelling, it should be sent for microbiological analysis (in a
plain sterile pot and in blood culture bottles to increase the success
rate of culture) but biochemical tests are not necessary. If the fluid
is clear and does not have an offensive odour, it should be sent for
both microbiological and biochemical analysis and should still be
treated as infected if the pH is less than 7.2 or the LDH is greater
than 1000 IU/l. Treatment is prompt closed drainage using an
intercostal drain, coupled with intravenous antibiotics. Empyema
often forms complex, loculated collections which are difficult to
drain adequately. Fibrinolytic agents, instilled via the drain, are
sometimes used in an attempt to break down loculations. Since the
mortality of empyema is high, a referral to thoracic surgeons
should be made early for patients in whom drainage is incomplete.

CHAPTER 5 – ANSWERS

Answer 2

(a) (i) Obstructive sleep apnoea/hypopnoea syndrome (OSAHS)

     (ii) Excessive daytime sleepiness
Poor concentration
Snoring   *(4 marks)*

(b) Hypertension
Cardiovascular disease
Stroke
Type II respiratory failure
Cor pulmonale
Industrial and road traffic accidents   *(3 marks)*

(c) Obtain adequate history, from both patient and partner, especially of sleeping habits
Examine, especially nasal patency, mouth, oropharynx and neck circumference
Arrange limited sleep study/polysomnography/ overnight pulse oximetry to confirm diagnosis
Treat with nocturnal continuous positive airways pressure (CPAP)   *(3 marks)*

Comment

Obstructive sleep apnoea/hypopnoea syndrome (OSAHS) is caused by occlusion of the upper airway as a result of reduced muscle tone during deep sleep. Transient arousal ensues, the airway musculature regains normal tone, the airway opens and breathing resumes. After a short while, the patient descends once again into deep sleep, the airway occludes, and the cycle repeats itself. The syndrome thus causes repeated interruptions to the normal sleeping pattern, leading to daytime hypersomnolence, abnormal release of stress hormones during sleep, and an increased risk of type II respiratory failure. Patients themselves may or may not be aware of snoring but their partners often report being frightened by the frequent prolonged pauses in breathing, or having to sleep in a different room to escape the noise.

Treatment of OSAHS starts with advice to lose weight and to avoid alcohol, sedative medication and smoking. Most sufferers also require continuous positive airways pressure (CPAP) to maintain airway patency, although patients with co-existing type II respiratory failure may be better treated with bi-level ventilation. Initiation of non-invasive ventilation requires skill and sensitivity from the clinician and sleep technician, and determination on the part of the patient. Intra-oral devices are available for patients who are unable to tolerate it. The role of surgery in the treatment of OSAHS in adults remains the subject of controversy.

Answer 3

(a) Spontaneous secondary left-sided pneumothorax

(1 mark)

(b) (i) Tension pneumothorax
    (ii) Tachypnoea
         Cyanosis
         Tracheal deviation (away from the pneumothorax)
         Tachycardia
         Hypotension
         Elevated jugular venous pressure
         Sweating *(4 marks)*

(c) Urgently:
   • Administer high-flow oxygen
   • Insert cannula into the second intercostal space, in the mid-clavicular line
   • Insert intercostal drain into the pleural space, through the fourth or fifth intercostal space in the mid-axillary line, and connect to an underwater seal.
   Once tension is relieved and the intercostal drain is bubbling, remove cannula from second intercostal space and arrange chest radiograph.
   Admit to hospital.
   Remove chest drain when it stops bubbling.
   Repeat chest radiograph. *(5 marks)*

Comment

Spontaneous pneumothorax is termed primary if it occurs in an otherwise healthy individual and secondary if the patient has pre-existing lung disease. Primary pneumothorax occurs more commonly in tall, rather than short, individuals, and both primary and secondary pneumothorax are much more common in smokers than in non-smokers. Tension pneumothorax is a rare complication, the risk being greater when pneumothorax occurs as a result of positive pressure ventilation or trauma.

Uncomplicated spontaneous pneumothorax may be treated conservatively if small (<2 cm rim between lung margin and chest wall on PA chest radiograph) and if there is minimal or no breathlessness. Inhalation of high-concentration oxygen increases by up to fourfold the rate of reabsorption of air from the pleural cavity. Aspiration is appropriate for larger volumes or for patients experiencing more than minimal breathlessness. If the lung is not successfully re-expanded by adequate (>2.5 l) aspiration, an intercostal drain is inserted and connected to an underwater seal. The integrity of the underwater seal, and hence the safety of the patient, depends on the bottle being kept upright and below the level of the patient's chest. The drain bubbles as air is forced out along the tube during expiration. Thus, if the lung is successfully re-expanded and the leak is closed, the drain stops bubbling but continues to swing with respiration. A non-bubbling, non-swinging drain is blocked or kinked. Patients whose drains continue to bubble after 48 h have persistent leaks and should be referred to a respiratory physician for consideration of use of vacuum or referral for thoracic surgery.

Tension pneumothorax is a medical emergency that, if not recognised and treated immediately, results rapidly in cardiorespiratory collapse and death. It is the only condition where intercostal drainage should precede imaging. The dramatic clinical signs are listed above; breath sounds may be reduced on the side of the pneumothorax at first but the chest quickly becomes silent in the absence of effective treatment. The first step is to insert a cannula, usually a 16G or 18G intravenous catheter, into the second intercostal space in the mid-clavicular line. A satisfying hiss of released air should ensue, confirming the diagnosis and treating it simultaneously. A formal intercostal drain should then be inserted and connected to an underwater seal, prior to arranging a chest radiograph.

Answer 4

(a) Tuberculosis
Pneumonia
Pulmonary embolism/infarction
Bronchogenic carcinoma
Metastatic malignancy
Rheumatoid disease
Systemic lupus erythematosus
Pancreatitis
Subphrenic abscess
Hepatic cirrhosis
Dressler's syndrome
Pleural endometriosis
Trauma (haemothorax, chylothorax)   *(3 marks)*

(b)

Macroscopic inspection (at bedside)	Clear/blood-stained, no foul odour
Cytology	Positive diagnosis of mesothelioma in a low proportion of cases
Protein	> 30 g/l, ie exudate
Lactate dehydrogenase (LDH)	Greater than two-thirds of the upper limit of normal for serum LDH, ie exudate
pH	< 7.6
Gram stain, culture & sensitivity, acid & alcohol-fast bacilli stain & culture	No organisms

(4 marks)

(c) CT thorax with contrast
CT-guided or ultrasound-guided percutaneous needle
biopsy
Video-assisted thorascopic surgery (VATS) procedure
with biopsy   *(3 marks)*

Comment

For the purposes of diagnosis, pleural effusions are classified as
transudate (protein < 30 g/l) or **exudate** (protein > 30 g/l). The
fluid protein value may be difficult to interpret if it is close to the
cut-off value, or if the serum protein level is abnormal, so Light's
criteria (see Table) may also be applied.

Pleural fluid is an exudate if any of the following criteria are met:

- The fluid protein level is greater than half the serum protein level
- The fluid LDH level is greater than 0.6 times the measured
  serum LDH level
- The fluid LDH level is greater than two-thirds the upper limit of
  normal for serum LDH.

Table: Light's criteria
Causes of pleural effusion are listed in the Table below. Conditions
which result in transudative effusions are often obvious on clinical
assessment, allowing pleural aspiration to be avoided unless the
effusion does not resolve with treatment of the underlying cause.

- **Transudate**
  - Congestive cardiac failure
  - Hypoalbuminaemia:
    - hepatic cirrhosis
    - nephrotic syndrome
    - severe malnutrition
    - severe systemic illness
  - Peritoneal dialysis
  - Pulmonary embolism
  - Hypothyroidism
  - Superior vena caval obstruction
  - Ovarian hyperstimulation
  - Meigs' syndrome

- **Exudate:**
  - Malignancy:
    ○ pleural
    ○ bronchial, by direct spread or metastasis
    ○ pericardial
    ○ other metastatic tumours, particularly breast & colon
    ○ lymphoma
  - Pneumonia
  - Tuberculosis
  - Pulmonary embolism
  - Rheumatoid disease
  - Systemic lupus erythematosus
  - Pancreatitis
  - Sub-phrenic abscess
  - Dressler's syndrome
  - Benign asbestos-related effusion
  - Yellow nail syndrome

Table: Causes of pleural effusion

Mesothelioma is a malignant tumour which occurs in individuals exposed to asbestos. There is a latent period of up to 40 years between exposure to asbestos fibres and development of disease. Typical features include:

- Dyspnoea secondary to large pleural effusion
- Chest pain, characteristically continuous, rather than pleuritic, because it arises from local invasion
- Weight loss
- Finger clubbing

It is often difficult to confirm a clinical diagnosis of mesothelioma prior to necropsy because mesothelioma deposits promote a dense fibrotic reaction, reducing the likelihood of positive pleural fluid cytology and of biopsying malignant tissue. In practice, when the diagnosis is suspected, an attempt at CT-guided percutaneous biopsy is usually made. If this is unsuccessful, a video-assisted thoroscopic surgery (VATS) procedure is performed by thoracic surgeons, allowing direct visualisation of the pleura, directly observed biopsy, complete drainage of any residual effusion, and talc pleurodesis (to prevent reaccumulation of the effusion), all during the same procedure.

Answer 5

(a) To exclude a pneumothorax and consolidation/lobar collapse   *(2 marks)*

(b) FBC; ABGs; PEFR; blood cultures; sputum culture
                                                         (3 marks)

(c) (i) Speech, pulse, respiratory rate, pulsus paradoxus, PEFR, oxygen saturation/ABGs, cyanosis
                                                         (2 marks)

(ii) Sit the patient upright
Oxygen (60%–100%) via mask; nebulised salbutamol and ipratropium
IV access
Oral or IV steroids
Oral or IV amoxicillin ± erythromycin   *(3 marks)*

Comment

Asthma is defined as a reversible obstruction of the intrathoracic airways, which varies in severity either spontaneously or with treatment.

It is a common respiratory disease, affecting between 5% and 10% of the population. Despite the advent of several therapeutic agents including the β2-adrenoceptor agonists, its mortality rate has not decreased in the last 30 years.

It is common to divide asthma into extrinsic or allergic, and intrinsic. Both groups exhibit bronchial hyperreactivity to various stimulants; these include the housedust mite, pollens, fungal spores, drugs, eg NSAIDs, and non-specific factors, such as emotional stress, exercise and cold air.

The severity of an acute exacerbation should be assessed by use of the following criteria:

	Mild to moderate	**Severe**
Pulse	Normal – tachycardia	Bradycardia
Blood pressure	Pulsus paradoxus	Maybe hypotensive
Respiratory rate	> 25/min	< 10/min
Speech	Normal – stilted sentences	Unable to talk
ABGs $p_a(O_2)$	Normal to 8.0 kPa	< 7.6–8.0 kPa
$p_a(CO_2)$	Normal or low (< 4.0 kPa)	> 6.0 kPa
PEFR	> 50% normal	< 30% normal
Cyanosis	Not present	Late/sinister sign

Patients with any combination of the severe signs should be considered for elective assisted ventilation.

See www.brit-thoracic.org.uk

Answer 6

(a) Atypical pneumonia *(1 mark)*

(b) *Mycoplasma pneumoniae*
Chlamydia psittaci
Legionella pneumophila
Coxiella burnetii *(4 marks)*

(c) (i) Haemolytic anaemia; depressed or normal WCC with abnormal differential count; thrombocytopenia
(ii) Hyponatraemia; raised urea and creatinine
(iii) Transient hepatitis
(iv) Type I respiratory failure
(v) Rising antibody titres; positive direct immunofluorescent stains *(5 marks)*

Comment

The term 'atypical pneumonia' seems to have lost favour recently, perhaps due to the increasing heterogeneity of the organisms included in this group. However, we feel the term is still useful in learning about this group as it prompts the student to think about why they are atypical. In particular they are atypical in their presentation, the clinical signs they produce, the investigations required to diagnose them and the atypical antibiotics required to break them. Some of these features are discussed below:

- **FBC** – *Mycoplasma* is commonly associated with a haemolytic anaemia with cold agglutinins. *Legionella* produces a relative lymphopaenia, whereas other organisms may depress the white cell count to subnormal levels. Many of the atypical organisms may also produce a thrombocytopenia
- **U&Es** – syndrome of inappropriate ADH (SIADH) producing a hyponatraemia is a feature of several atypicals, particularly *Legionella* infection. Dehydration, secondary to nausea and vomiting or diarrhoea, may cause mild prerenal impairment
- **LFTs** – a transient hepatitis is another common feature which may, in turn, be exacerbated by erythromycin
- **Skin** – generalised rashes are common but *Mycoplasma* may cause erythema multiforme and the Stevens–Johnson syndrome. *Chlamydia psittaci* may cause rose spots on the abdomen
- **CNS** – drowsiness and confusion may be features, as may depression. They may also present with a meningitic picture, as well as causing a meningo-encephalitis

Other features include diarrhoea and vomiting, pharyngitis and more unusually pericarditis, myocarditis and rarely *Coxiella*-associated endocarditis. The organisms are generally difficult to culture in the laboratory but are now more readily identifiable by use of direct immunofluorescent stains and specific antibodies. Treatment may include the use of erythromycin, tetracycline and rifampicin, but should always include antistreptococcal agents, as it is far more common, and can be fatal if untreated.

Answer 7

(a) A full respiratory and cardiovascular history
Previous medical history – particularly previous
whooping cough, measles, asthma, tuberculosis
Treatment history to exclude exacerbating drugs,
eg NSAIDs and β-blockers
Smoking history – duration, type, number/day
Occupational history – eg exposure to industrial dusts
Exposure to domestic animals and birds   *(5 marks)*

(b) Chest X-ray, PEFR, spirometery – before and after
nebuliser, ECG, ABGs   *(3 marks)*

(c) β2-agonists – salbutamol, terbutaline
Anticholinergics – long acting tiotropium
(ipratropium is still used in its nebulised form)
Theophylline – aminophylline
Steroids – inhaled, oral or intravenous   *(2 marks)*

Comment

Chronic obstructive pulmonary disease (COPD) is a progressive
illness caused by smoking. It is characterised by airflow
obstruction that is not fully reversible. The extent of airflow
obstruction is assessed by spirometry and expressed as a reduction
in the FEV_1/FVC ratio. Patients with COPD have classically been
divided into 'pink puffers' and the 'blue bloaters', suffering type I
and type II failure, respectively. Type I respiratory failure is defined
as hypoxia ($p_a(O_2) < 10.6$ kPa) associated with a normal or low
arterial carbon dioxide, ($p_a(CO_2) = 4.6$ kPa), whereas type II
failure is hypoxia associated with a raised arterial carbon dioxide
($p_a(CO_2) > 6.4$ kPa). Therapeutic agents such as β2-agonists,
anticholinergics, theophylline and steroids are often given with
subjective improvement, but no interventions other than cessation
of smoking and long-term oxygen therapy have any bearing on
prognosis. Patients qualify for long-term home oxygen by fulfilling
the following criteria, based on two sets of arterial blood gases and

spirometry, with the patient stable: $p_aO_2 < 7.3$ kPa; or $p_aO_2 > 8.0$ kPa with one or more of secondary polycythaemia, nocturnal hypoxaemia, peripheral oedema or pulmonary hypertension. Patients only gain mortality benefit from long-term oxygen if it is used for at least 15, and preferably 20, hours per day.

See www.brit-thoracic.org.uk/guidelines.html

Answer 8

(a)   Bronchogenic carcinoma   *(1 mark)*

(b)   CXR; sputum for cytology; bronchoscopy with
brushings and biopsy
CT scan of the thorax   *(3 marks)*

(c)   Chemotherapy is used alone or as an adjuvant to
surgery and/or radiotherapy
Surgery – may be curative; may be combined with
chemotherapy and radiotherapy
Radiotherapy – may be used as a monotherapy or in
combination. It is also used to palliate bony pain of
metastases and for recurrent haemoptysis
Palliative care involving specialist medical and nursing
staff should be considered in cases presenting with
advanced disease   *(6 marks)*

Comment

Bronchial carcinoma is the commonest malignancy in the Western world, with an annual mortality of 35 000 people in the UK alone. It affects three to four times as many men as women, but the female incidence continues to increase. In this case the diagnosis of carcinoma is the most likely, although pulmonary tuberculosis, bronchiectasis, lung abscess and the systemic vasculitides may all present in this way. The diagnosis may be inferred from a chest X-ray and confirmed by sputum cytology and bronchoscopy with bronchial washings and biopsy. CT scan of the thorax may be required to localise and stage the tumour. The therapeutic options include surgery, chemotherapy, radiotherapy and palliative care. Operative intervention is limited by the patient's respiratory reserve, the anatomical site and staging of the tumour. However, in non-small cell disease, it is potentially curative. In general, elderly patients do badly with surgery. Chemotherapy is principally used in small cell disease, where it is proven to improve prognosis. Combination therapy is now also used in advanced, inoperable non-small cell disease, but with little effect on long-term prognosis. Various combinations of chemotherapeutic agents are used, including adriamycin, methotrexate, cyclophosphamide and newer agents, including ifosfamide.

Answer 9

(a) Pulmonary embolism *(1 mark)*

(b) Recent long distance journey or prolonged period of immobility
Recent major surgery
Recent fracture – particularly pelvic and lower limb
Family history of coagulopathy or thromboembolic disease
Oral contraceptive pill and pregnancy
Coagulopathy – protein C and S, antithrombin III deficiency; anticardiolipin antibody; factor V Leiden mutation (the commonest of several recently elucidated gene mutations) *(3 marks)*

(c) (i) Investigations:
FBC, clotting screen
ABGs
CXR
ECG
CTPA or VQ scan *(3 marks)*

(ii) Therapeutic management:
       Sit the patient upright; oxygen via a mask
       IV access
       Analgesia
       Subcutaneous LMWH e.g. enoxaparin 1mg/kg
       bd or 1.5mg/kg od
       On confirmation of the diagnosis, six months'
       therapy with warfarin, maintaining the INR
       between 2 and 3
       Address and treat underlying risk factors
                                        (3 marks)

Comment

One should always have a low threshold for treating a patient for pulmonary embolism, particularly in the presence of any combination of risk factors. (A second embolism could be fatal!) Initial investigations may often produce non-specific results but add to clinical suspicions:

- **FBC** – this may show polycythaemia, thrombocytosis or an abnormal white cell count suggestive of a haematological malignancy.
- **Clotting screen** – in cases where there is no identifiable risk factors this should include protein C and S, and antithrombin III levels, and anticardiolipin antibody. Recently, factor V Leiden mutation has been identified as an important cause in this subgroup.
- **ABGs** – show type I respiratory failure, often with hypocapnia.
- **ECG** – the principal abnormality is a sinus tachycardia, but in larger PEs a right ventricular strain pattern may occur, with a dominant R wave in V1 and V2. The classical pattern of $S_1Q_3T_3$ is rarely seen, but should always be sought.
- **CXR** – may be normal; however, it may produce a wedge shadow or oligaemic areas. It is also necessary to exclude pneumonias and pneumothoraces, which may present in a similar manner.

CTPA has largely superceded V/Q Scanning in most centres, except in sub-acute presentations where small sub-segmental pulmonary emboli are suspected.

Answer 10

(a) Erythema nodosum
Keratoconjunctivitis sicca   *(2 marks)*

(b) Skin involvement – lupus pernio, sarcoid infiltration of the skin
Neurological – peripheral neuropathy, cranial nerve palsies, aseptic meningitis, hypopituitarism
Eyes – anterior uveitis, choroidoretinitis
'Sicca syndrome' – infiltration of the salivary and lacrimal glands
Joints – arthralgia
Hepatosplenomegaly
Renal – renal stones, hypercalciuria and associated nephrocalcinosis
Lymphadenopathy
Cardiomyopathy, cor pulmonale and conduction system disease   *(3 marks)*

(c) CXR
Transbronchial biopsy and broncho-alveolar lavage
Liver biopsy
Formal respiratory function tests
Serum angiotensin converting enzyme (ACE)
Kveim test
Tuberculin test   *(5 marks)*

Comment

Sarcoidosis is a common, multisystem granulomatous disorder, which presents usually between 25 and 35 years of age. It is more common in women and in certain racial groups. It has a more severe presentation and malignant progression in Black compared to White races. Clinically it is characterised by pulmonary infiltration, skin and eye involvement, and on chest X-ray by bilateral hilar lymphadenopathy. The pathogenesis and aetiology remain unclear. It is thought that environmental agents trigger an abnormal immune response, with helper T-cells at its centre. These cause the formation of non-caseating granulomata, which in turn leads to a fibrotic response in the affected tissues. The course and prognosis of the disease can be inferred by the mode of presentation. Acute onset in young adults, with associated erythema nodosum, usually signifies a self-limiting disorder. Later, more insidious onset in middle age leads to a progressive disorder, with multisystem fibrosis.

Pulmonary sarcoid is classified by the radiological changes seen on chest X-ray, into four stages:

- Stage 0 (clear CXR)
- Stage 1 (bilateral hilar and mediastinal lymphadenopathy)
- Stage 2 (stage 1 + associated pulmonary infiltration)
- Stage 3 (pulmonary infiltration without hilar lymphadenopathy).

No therapy has as yet been shown to influence the progression of the disease. Steroids are recommended in stages 2 and 3 of the pulmonary disease, and for eye and cardiac involvement. Chloroquine is also used in therapy, as are NSAIDs.

Answer 11

(a) Cystic fibrosis *(1 mark)*

(b) Pancreatic endocrine involvement leading to diabetes mellitus
Pancreatic exocrine involvement leading to steatorrhoea and malabsorption
Bronchiectasis *(3 marks)*

(c)   Nutritional support with pancreatic enzyme
supplements and regular dietetic review
Diabetic education and insulin therapy
Daily chest physiotherapy, which may be performed by
relatives
Rapid and appropriate treatment of infective
exacerbations
Sputum viscosity reduction
Genetic counselling of parents and patient
Consider for heart lung transplant   *(6 marks)*

Comment

Cystic fibrosis is an autosomal recessive disorder, whose gene
mutation has now been localised to the long arm of chromosome 7.
The protein encoded in this region is called the cystic fibrosis
transmembrane regulator. With improvements in physiotherapy,
antimicrobials and nutritional support, life expectancy in this
group has now improved to 30–40 years. Patients usually present in
childhood with recurrent pulmonary symptoms, cystic fibrosis
being the principal cause of chronic suppurative lung disease in this
age group. They may also present with constipation or even acute
obstruction due to meconium ileus equivalent (MIE), meconium
ileus being a presenting feature in the neonate.

Males are invariably infertile due to the absence of development of
the vas deferens and the epididymis, but females are able to
conceive providing the secondary effects of the illness, such as
malnutrition, can be prevented or minimised.

The diagnosis is confirmed from the family history, a sodium
sweat test and chromosomal analysis. Treatment should be
instituted and followed up in a regional or area centre of
excellence, so that complications of the disease are rapidly
identified and minimised. Pseudomonal chest infection is the
main cause of exacerbation of the chest symptoms and is often
the cause of death. Providing the patient's health can be
stabilised, there is 65% survival at three years and 50% survival at
five years. In severe cases a heart–lung transplant remains the

only viable option at the present time. Gene manipulation may offer a future cure.

Answer 12

(a) Idiopathic pulmonary fibrosis (previously termed cryptogenic fibrosing alveolitis) *(1 mark)*

(b) Rheumatoid arthritis, systemic lupus erythematosus
Progressive systemic sclerosis
Inflammatory bowel disease
Primary biliary cirrhosis *(3 marks)*

(c) CXR – lower zone fibrosis
ABGs – type I respiratory failure
Lung function tests – restrictive lung defect, with a reduced transfer coefficient
High resolution CT scan of the thorax – confirms the distribution of the fibrosis *(6 marks)*

Comment

Idiopathic pulmonary fibrosis (previously termed cryptogenic fibrosing alveolitis) is defined as fibrosis of the distal airways, in the absence of any identifiable cause. It may present at any age but is most commonly seen in the sixth and seventh decades. It has an equal sex distribution but its prevalence is increased amongst smokers. It is associated with several immune-mediated disorders, but its own aetiology remains unclear. Patients present with progressive exertional dyspnoea, associated with a non-productive cough. Haemoptysis is a sinister sign and should alert the physician to the possibility of an underlying malignancy, which is 10 to 15 times more common than in the general population. Clubbing occurs in 70%–80% of cases and many also have fine inspiratory crepitations, principally heard at the lung bases. In the more severe cases, there may also be cyanosis and signs of cor pulmonale. The diagnosis is confirmed by lung function tests, high-resolution CT scan of the thorax, and bronchoscopy and broncho-alveolar lavage. Arterial blood gases show type I respiratory failure, the hypoxia classically worsening on exertion. Since the disease is idiopathic, there is no specific treatment. Various new regimes are under investigation, including high-dose steroids, and immunosuppressants, such as azathioprine, cyclophosphamide and ciclosporin, but the prognosis remains poor with a 50% mortality rate at five years.

Answer 13

(a) The pneumoconioses
Silicosis
Berylliosis   *(3 marks)*

(b) His shortness of breath is caused by pulmonary fibrosis secondary to asbestosis. The haemoptysis is secondary to a bronchogenic carcinoma   *(2 marks)*

(c) Pleural thickening
Calcified pleural and diaphragmatic plaques
Lower zone fibrosis initially, which may become more widespread
Advanced cases may show signs of 'honeycombing', with a hazy irregular cardiac silhouette
Bronchial carcinoma and associated signs, eg hilar lymphadenopathy   *(5 marks)*

Comment

Chronic exposure to asbestos, in particular crocidolite (blue asbestos), causes a chronic pulmonary fibrotic disorder, asbestosis. This classically affects the lower zones of the lungs, unlike the other pneumoconioses, which affect the apices. (The radiological findings of pleural and diaphragmatic plaques only imply previous asbestos exposure and the patient should not be labelled as having asbestosis.)

Asbestos exposure is the principal risk factor in the development of mesothelioma, which may be pleural, peritoneal and more rarely pericardial. Both the duration and the concentration of fibre exposure are important in the development of the tumour.

CHAPTER 5 – ANSWERS

Classically the tumour manifests itself 30–40 years after the initial exposure. There is currently no effective treatment and the prognosis remains poor, with a median survival of 18 months. Smoking has a synergistic effect with asbestos fibres and increases the risk of developing a bronchogenic carcinoma almost 100 times that of a non-smoker never exposed to asbestos.

Asbestosis and the other pneumoconioses are industrial notifiable diseases in the UK, for which the patient and their families are eligible for compensation.

Answer 14

(a) Farmer's lung; this is an example of extrinsic allergic alveolitis *(2 marks)*

(b)

Agents	Sources
Aspergillus spp	Whisky maltings, vegetable compost
Penicillium spp	Cheese, wood, cork
Birds	Feathers and excreta

(4 marks)

(c) He should be advised that chronic exposure may cause a progressive lung condition with fibrosis, causing increasing shortness of breath and disability. He should minimise exposure to precipitating agents by changing his work duties, using an industrial respirator to filter out dusts, and improve the ventilation in the working environment; the use of oral and inhaled steroids is beneficial in an acute attack *(4 marks)*

Comment

Extrinsic allergic alveolitis is the term given to the group of pulmonary disorders caused by hypersensitivity to inhaled dusts. They are alternatively termed hypersensitivity pneumonitis, as the resulting inflammatory process occurs in all of the distal airways involved in gaseous exchange, and not just the alveoli.

Clinically the disease is divided into acute and chronic forms. In the **acute form** the sensitised patient, ie someone previously exposed to the causative dust, presents several hours after a further exposure, with acute dyspnoea and a non-productive cough. They often complain of an associated flu-like illness. Occasionally, the patient may present with a wheeze and a productive cough predominating. In the **chronic form** there is progressive pulmonary fibrosis, principally in the apices of the lungs. As the diseases progresses the fibrosis becomes more widespread and this leads to secondary pulmonary hypertension and cor pulmonale.

Management is based on excluding or reducing exposure to the causative agent. However, patients often chose to continue exposure, eg pigeon fanciers. In industrial cases the patient is eligible for compensation if the chronic form of the disease develops, but many patients with the acute form choose to continue working, with few progressing to the chronic, symptomatic disease. In these cases inhaled or oral steroids are used in acute on chronic episodes; however, the use of long-term steroids in the chronic disease has not been shown to influence the prognosis.

Answer 15

(a) Adult respiratory distress syndrome (ARDS)   *(1 mark)*

(b) CXR appearances of pulmonary oedema
Hypoxaemia ($p_a(O_2) < 6.7$ kPa), on 60%–100% inspired oxygen   *(2 marks)*

(c) (i) FBC, U&Es, glucose, clotting screen including FDPs and D-dimer, group and save
Blood cultures
ABGs
CXR
ECG
MSU or CSU   *(3 marks)*

(ii) Management is based on the haemodynamic status of the patient:

With adequate blood pressure – sit the patient upright

If the patient is shocked – start colloid infusion

Patient will require central venous access and inotrope support, therefore more senior help should be sought immediately

In either case – IV access 60%–100% oxygen via a mask

IV broad spectrum antibiotics and diuretics

(4 marks)

Comment

ARDS should always be suspected in any patient with acute respiratory failure and any predisposing factors, such as:

- Hypovolaemia/haemorrhage
- Sepsis – this is implicated in 80% of patients
- Trauma – this includes burns
- Thrombotic, fat and amniotic emboli
- Aspiration pneumonia and drowning
- Inhalation of smoke and noxious gases
- Drug overdose – barbiturates, NSAIDs, heroin
- Metabolic disturbances – uraemia, ketoacidosis

ARDS has several diagnostic criteria:

- CXR – the radiographic changes vary from isolated areas to diffuse alveolar infiltration, consistent with pulmonary oedema; they often correlate poorly with the clinical condition of the patient
- Hypoxaemia – the $p_a(O_2)$ must be < 6.7 kPa on 60%–100% inspired oxygen
- Reduced lung compliance – this is confirmed on ventilating the patient
- Exudative pulmonary oedema
- PCWP < 18 mmHg – this excludes cardiogenic oedema, where the PCWP is > 18 mmHg
- Pulmonary hypertension > 30/15 mmHg

Treatment should include appropriate management of the underlying cause, correction of any specific metabolic disturbances and assisted ventilation in an intensive care unit. No specific treatment has been shown to influence the prognosis. Failure to recognise and treat the condition leads to rapid deposition of proteinaceous and hyaline material leading to alveolar collapse and, within 48 hours, irreversible interstitial fibrosis.

Cardiology

Answer 1

(a) Acute coronary syndrome: unstable angina
(crescendo angina) *(2 marks)*

(b) Oxygen
Aspirin 300 mg po
Clopidogrel 300 mg po
Glyceryl trinitrate or isosorbide dinitrate IV infusion
Low-molecular-weight heparin, eg enoxaparin,
dalteparin
Beta-blocker, eg metoprolol or bisporolol
(which have largely superceded atenolol);
carvedilol is another drug which may be considered
Diamorphine if pain not rapidly controlled *(4 marks)*

(c) Troponin I is a cardiac-specific regulatory sub-unit of
the contractile apparatus of striated muscle
Injury to cardiac muscle results in its release into the
circulation
This patient's result indicates that no irreversible
ischaemic damage has occurred
Despite this, the reversible ST depression indicates he is
at high risk of a subsequent coronary event and so
should undergo urgent coronary angiography with a
view to revascularisation (coronary artery bypass
grafting or percutaneous coronary angioplasty and
stent) *(4 marks)*

Comment

The term 'acute coronary syndrome' encompasses the range of clinical presentations arising from an acute reduction in, or cessation of, coronary artery blood flow. These comprise new-onset angina, unstable angina, non-ST elevation myocardial infarction and myocardial infarction causing ST elevation or new-onset bundle branch block. Unstable angina is the term for ischaemic discomfort that occurs at rest or on minimal exertion. The characteristic clinical features are of tight, central chest pain, that is often described as crushing, like a vice, or like a band tightening around the chest. The pain is associated with sweating, dyspnoea and pallor. Unstable angina may occur with or without pre-existing stable (ie exertional) angina but, if the preceding history is of worsening severity of previously exertional symptoms, this is known as 'crescendo angina'. Emergency treatments for unstable angina include oxygen, anti-platelet agents, low-molecular-weight heparin and vasodilators. Glycoprotein IIb/IIIa inhibitors (abciximab, eptifibatide, tirofiban) are licensed for use in unstable angina but their use is generally confined to patients with continuing ST depression despite initial treatment. Such patients should also undergo urgent coronary angiography with a view to revascularisation.

Troponin T and troponin I are undetectable in the blood of healthy individuals but are released by myocardium undergoing profound ischaemia or infarction. Diagnostic concentrations are reached 12 hours after an acute event. Troponin assays thus provide a sensitive and specific indication of whether myocardial damage has occurred. Along with measurement of cardiac enzymes (CK-MB, LDH), serial ECGs and, in the post-acute setting, stress-testing or perfusion-scanning, they are used to predict the risk of a subsequent coronary event occurring.

Answer 2

(a) Third-degree atrioventricular block with a proximal
ventricular escape rhythm   *(2 marks)*

(b) Beta-blockers, eg metoprolol, atenolol, bisoprolol,
propranolol
Non-dihydropyridine calcium-channel blockers:
verapamil, diltiazem
Anti-arrhythmics: amiodarone, flecainide   *(4 marks)*

(c) Conservative management in a monitored, coronary
care environment
Atropine 600 µg IV
External pacing (with sedation)
Temporary ventricular pacing   *(4 marks)*

Comment

A classification of atrioventricular block is given in the table
below. Atrioventricular block occurring in association with
inferior myocardial infarction usually resolves within seven to ten
days, whereas, in the setting of anterior myocardial infarction, it is
usually permanent.

In this case, the ventricular rate and the QRS-complex
morphology indicate that the escape rhythm arises above the
bifurcation of the bundle of His. A more distal escape rhythm
results in a broad (longer duration) QRS complex and a slower
rate. The more distal the escape rhythm, the greater the risk of
asystolic arrest. Since temporary ventricular pacing is associated
with a considerable risk of infection, its use in this case should be
reserved for progression to a more distal escape rhythm despite
atropine treatment, or for the development of haemodynamic
decompensation. External pacing is extremely uncomfortable
and so is only used, with sedation, in the treatment of life-
threatening haemodynamic compromise until a temporary
pacing wire can be inserted.

Table: Classification of atrioventricular block

First degree	Prolongation of PR interval beyond 0.20 seconds
Second degree	Intermittent failure of conduction across the atrioventricular node
Type I (Wenckebach phenomenon)	Gradually increasing PR interval in successive beats until a non-conducted P-wave occurs. Occasionally a non-pathological finding in healthy young adults
Type II	Intermittent failure of P-wave conduction without preceding gradual PR interval prolongation. May occur sporadically or at regular intervals, eg 2:1 or 3:1 conduction
Third degree	Complete dissociation between atrial electrical activity and ventricular contraction

Answer 3

(a) Acute idiopathic pericarditis
Coxsackieviruses
Echoviruses
Mumps
Rubella
Hepatitis B
Influenza   *(4 marks)*

(b) Widespread ST elevation, typically saddle-shaped
Variable T-wave flattening and inversion over next few weeks
Eventual complete resolution   *(3 marks)*

(c) Acute myocardial infarction
Dressler's syndrome
Post-cardiotomy syndrome
Intra-pericardial haemorrhage
Renal failure
Autoimmune connective tissue diseases and vasculitides
Neoplasia
Mediastinal irradiation   *(3 marks)*

CHAPTER 6 – ANSWERS

Comment

Acute idiopathic pericarditis is a clinical diagnosis based on the characteristic pain, pericardial rub and ECG changes. Viral serology is frequently negative.

Echocardiography is useful to look for a co-existing pericardial effusion that, if present, should be monitored to ensure that it does not enlarge to cause tamponade. Complete resolution is the rule. The only treatment required for uncomplicated cases is analgesia, usually with non-steroidal anti-inflammatories (NSAIDs).

Pericarditis may also occur as a result of bacterial infection, including by *Mycobacterium tuberculosis*, especially in immunocompromised patients.

Myocardial infarction, particularly when transmural, may cause an acute pericarditis within the first two to three days. This situation is associated with accentuation of typical post-MI ECG changes, and should be differentiated from Dressler's syndrome. The latter condition is an acute febrile illness, accompanied by pericarditis, that occurs two to four weeks after myocardial infarction. Post-cardiotomy syndrome presents in a similar fashion and the two conditions are likely to share an immune-mediated aetiology.

Answer 4

(a) Atrial flutter with 2:1 block
Atrial tachycardia
AV nodal re-entry tachycardia
Sinus tachycardia   *(4 marks)*

(b) Alcohol excess
Caffeine excess
Hypertension
Thyrotoxicosis
Pulmonary embolism
Sepsis
Hypovolaemia
Anaemia *(3 marks)*

(c) If atrial flutter waves are not obvious, adenosine will reveal them but will not terminate atrial flutter.
Amiodarone intravenously (300 mg over 30 min then 1200 mg per 24 h) is the usual first choice.
If this fails, DC cardioversion is effective.
If arrhythmia is long-standing, anticoagulate before chemical or electrical cardioversion. *(3 weeks)*

Comment

Regular tachycardias are classified according to the duration of the QRS complex (see Table). In narrow-complex tachycardia, vagal manoeuvres and/or adenosine are useful. They cause transient AV nodal block, terminating some arrhythmias (particularly AV nodal re-entry tachycardia) and revealing the nature of underlying atrial activity where cardioversion does not occur. The short half-life of adenosine (usually just a few seconds but prolonged in patients taking dipyridamole) makes it relatively safe and allows use of a second drug if necessary. If cardioversion does not occur with a second drug, it is wiser to use synchronised DC shock (under general anaesthesia or deep sedation) than additional antiarrhythmic drugs, since the risk of proarrhythmic side-effects with drug combinations is considerable.

Narrow QRS complex regular tachycardias:

Sinus tachycardia	Rate rarely >150 beats/min except during exercise	Treat underlying cause, eg sepsis, anaemia
Atrial flutter	Atrial flutter occurs at 300 beats/min but conduction block usually occurs, commonly 2:1, resulting in a ventricular rate of 150 per min	Neither adenosine nor vagal manoeuvres terminate atrial flutter but either will reveal saw-tooth flutter waves if doubt exists over diagnosis. Amiodarone cardioverts
Atrial tachycardia	May occur in digoxin toxicity. Rate of 120–250 per min. P waves visible, approximately normal appearance	Amiodarone or verapamil cardiovert. In digoxin toxicity, correct hypokalaemia and consider beta-blockade and digoxin-specific antibody fragments
Atrio-ventricular nodal re-entry tachycardia	Rate of 140–220 per min. P waves virtually invisible	Vagal manoeuvres, adenosine or verapamil cardiovert
Atrio-ventricular re-entry tachycardia	Rate of 140–220 per min. Retrograde P waves may be visible during tachycardia. Delta wave and short PR interval may be visible on sinus rhythm ECG	Vagal manoeuvres, adenosine or verapamil cardiovert

Broad QRS complex tachycardias:

Ventricular tachycardia	Rate >120 per min	Lignocaine, amiodarone or DC cardioversion
Torsades de pointes	Continuously varying QRS axis. Associated with prolongation of the QT interval	Magnesium sulphate infusion
Supraventricular tachycardia with aberrant conduction	If there is any doubt over the diagnosis, it is safer to treat a broad-complex tachycardia as VT. (Verapamil causes haemodynamic collapse and sudden death in VT)	

Answer 5

(a) (i) Acute myocardial infarction *(1 mark)*

    (ii) Risk factors:
Smoking
Previous history of IHD or stroke
Known diabetes mellitus, hypertension, PVD
Family history of IHD or stroke
Alcohol excess *(2 marks)*

(b) Aspirin and clopidogrel
Beta-blockers, eg atenolol, metoprolol, bisoprolol, carvedilol
ACEIs, eg captopril, enalapril, ramipril, lisinopril, perindopril
Thrombolytic agents, eg streptokinase, tPA
Lipid-lowering agents, eg pravastatin, simvastatin
Insulin
LMWH *(3 marks)*

(c) History:

Need to clarify site, character, time of onset, duration, intensity/severity, radiation of the pain exacerbating/relieving factors, risk factors, present medications, contraindications to thrombolysis

Examination:

Assess haemodynamic status, signs of cardiac failure, presence of murmurs, signs of hyperlipidaemia, PVD, hypertension, diabetes mellitus

Investigations:

FBC, U&Es, glucose, lipids, cardiac enzymes (troponin)

CXR

ECG

Treatment:

Sit the patient upright

IV access

Oxygen via a mask

Analgesia

Aspirin 300 mg (stat)

Confirm diagnosis based on history, examination, ECG, and cardiac enzymes

If no contraindications give thrombolysis

In next 24–48 hours consider secondary prophylaxis, ie ACEIs and/or β-blockers; address all risk factors; education re: lifestyle by specialist nurse practitioners *(4 marks)*

Comment

Within the last 15 years, several worldwide mega trials, in particular the ISIS series and GUSTO, have dramatically changed the treatment and prognosis of acute myocardial infarction. Aspirin, thrombolysis and insulin have all been shown to improve prognosis in the first 24 hours, and secondary prophylaxis with ACEIs, β-blockers and simvastatin have improved post-infarction morbidity and survival. Recently, larger tertiary referral hospitals have set up 24 hour centres for patients with acute infarcts and this has meant many patients receive definitive, angiographic guided intervention (stenting and angioplasty) within hours of the onset of their pain. In turn this has led to a reduction in the previously common post infarct complications and patients are now able to leave hospital within 48 hours of admission.

Admission of a patient with a confirmed infarct can be divided into two phases: the acute phase or first 24 hours, and the secondary phase, which incorporates the rest of the admission and beyond.

Acute phase

- Diagnosis is confirmed by history, examination, and investigations
- Sit the patient upright, oxygen via mask
- IV access
- Analgesia – initially sublingual or buccal nitrates

If this has poor effect, IV diamorphine with IV anti-emetic is given (drugs should not be administered im as this will affect the enzyme results)

- Stat dose of aspirin 300 mg

After their initial aspirin (given by the paramedical team aboard the ambulance) patients are then divided and classified by their ECG findings. Patients with ST elevation MIs (STEMIs) may be transferred directly to an angiography suite and further intervention guided by the angiographic findings. If this facility is not available, thrombolysis with tPA is given for patients with no contra-indications.

In those Non-STEMI or unstable angina (sub-divided by the troponin result), patients are given LMWH, clopidogrel and aspirin, and may be considered for a GIIb/IIIa receptor antagonist (although in most centres this is still not used routinely.)

(The secondary phase of treatment is the same in both groups of patients and dealt with in the next question.)

Answer 6

(a) Aspirin
ACE inhibitor
Lipid-lowering agent, e.g. simvastatin
Oral hypoglycaemic, eg gliclazide *(4 marks)*

(b) Dietician – needs advice on low-cholesterol, diabetic diet *(1 mark)*

(c) Address all risk factors – hyperlipidaemia, diabetes, smoking, alcohol excess, obesity, lack of exercise
Patient education about prognosis and lifestyle
Education about further angina, the possible need for antianginal therapy and the use of GTN tablets or spray; if regular chest pain, he will require further investigation, which includes exercise stress testing and possible coronary angiography *(5 marks)*

Comment

All patients suffering from ischaemic heart disease should be on some form of secondary prophylaxis. Patients with no contraindications should be on low-dose aspirin, 75 mg per day and/or clopidogrel 75 mg per day, and, depending on their left ventricular function, a β-blocker or an ACE inhibitor, and in some cases both. Left ventricular function is assessed clinically, by the presence or absence of basal crepitations; radiographically, by the CXR signs of pulmonary oedema and cardiomegaly; and objectively by echocardiography. ACE inhibitors stop 'ventricular remodelling', which occurs after an ischaemic insult, thus reducing 'dysfunctional contractility' of the affected myocardium. Beta-blockers reduce the myocardial contractility and therefore reduce the demand for increased blood supply. Recent work has shown that ACE inhibitors improve the prognosis in all patients, irrespective of their left ventricular function, and that in patients with mild to moderate left ventricular impairment, beta-blockers should now be given with or without an ACE inhibitor. In practice, however, most patients are placed on only one of these agents.

On-going anginal symptoms require medical intervention with anti-anginal therapy. Beta-blockers are the first-line choice, if not contraindicated, then, depending on symptoms, oral nitrates, calcium-channel blockers and potassium channel activators can be added. A newer anti-anginal, ivabradine, has recently been introduced which acts on I_f channels in the sino-atrial node. This causes bradycardia and thus ivabradine should not be used with beta blockers and with caution with other rate limiting drugs. If medical therapy fails to control anginal symptoms further investigations should be initiated, starting with an exercise stress test. The patient must be made aware that, depending on the results of this test, they may require coronary angiography, angioplasty or possible bypass surgery.

Answer 7

(a) Beta-blockers and calcium-channel blockers *(2 marks)*

(b) The radiological features include:
Cardiomegaly, upper lobe blood diversion, Kerley B lines, pleural effusions, fluid in the horizontal fissure, and interstitial shadowing consistent with pulmonary oedema
Other findings may include:
Calcification of the heart valves
Left ventricular aneurysm *(4 marks)*

(c) Management should include:
Full history and examination to identify underlying risk factors and their associated signs

Investigations:
FBC, U&Es, glucose, lipids, TFTs
CXR
ECG
Echocardiogram
Address any underlying risk factors: stop smoking,
decrease alcohol excess, improve diet, weight loss if
appropriate – review by dietician, hypertension,
hyperlipidaemia, unstable angina
Increase exercise participation
Specific therapeutic agents – diuretics, ACE inhibitors,
digoxin, nitrates, others, eg hydralazine   *(4 marks)*

Comment

The prognosis in biventricular cardiac failure remains poor,
despite the introduction of new therapeutic agents such as ACE
inhibitors, spironolactone, cardio selective beta blockers and
carvedilol. As symptoms progress other medications including
nitrates, digoxin and vasodilators, such as hydralazine and
prazosin should be introduced. The one-year mortality rate is
approximately 50%. Ischaemic heart disease, hypertension and
idiopathic dilated cardiomyopathy remain by far the commonest
causes in the Western world. Others include:

- Cardiomyopathy (toxic, eg alcohol)
- Restrictive
- Hypertrophic
- Myocardial infiltration (fibrosis, sarcoidosis, amyloidosis,
  haemochromatosis)
- Valvular dysfunction (endocarditis, rheumatic valvular disease,
  congenital valvular disease)
- Chronic arrhythmia (brady and tachyarrhythmia)
- Drugs (β-blockers, NSAIDs, calcium-channel blockers)
- Systemic disease (acromegaly, thyroid disease, anaemia)

The management of heart failure must initially address any
underlying risk factors, associated disease, and improve the
patient's understanding of their condition.

First-line medications should include loop diuretics and ACE inhibitors, and then with symptom progression nitrates, digoxin and vasodilators, such as prazosin, should be introduced. Formal anticoagulation should also be considered, as this group are particularly at risk from DVT and left ventricular thrombus formation. Cardiac transplant, although offering a 'cure', remains limited due to lack of donor hearts and financial constraint. Transplant survival is estimated at 50% at five years. Trials with implantable mechanical pumps are underway.

See http://guidance.nice.org.uk/topic/cardiovascular

Answer 8

(a) (i) Atrial fibrillation *(1 mark)*

    (ii) Ischaemic heart disease – due to smoking and alcohol excess
Cardiomyopathy – due to alcohol excess or ischaemic heart disease *(2 marks)*

(b) Transient ischaemic attack *(2 marks)*

(c) History and examination – to assess risk factors and their associated signs in particular hypertension, cardiac murmurs, and cardiac failure
Investigations:
    FBC, U&Es, glucose, lipids, TFTs
    CXR
    ECG 24-hour tape
    Echocardiogram
Therapeutic management:
    Address underlying risk factors and associated disease
    Drugs – digoxin, amiodarone, sotalol
    Add aspirin 300 mg od in this case (alcohol excess precludes formal anticoagulation with warfarin)
    Consider synchronised DC cardioversion *(5 marks)*

Comment

Atrial fibrillation, particularly in its paroxysmal form, is associated with increased morbidity and mortality. Systemic emboli lead to TIAs, stroke, limb and mesenteric embolisation, all of which may be fatal. Once the diagnosis is confirmed, the aim of therapy is to cardiovert the patient back into sinus rhythm, which may be achieved either chemically with drugs or by synchronised DC cardioversion. If this is unachievable then control of the ventricular rate must be achieved by drug therapy. The patient should be anticoagulated with warfarin, with the INR kept between 2 and 3. If warfarin is contraindicated then aspirin should be considered. Once the patient has been anticoagulated for at least three weeks, synchronised DC cardioversion may be attempted. However, it is rarely used in patients with chronic organic heart disease or long-standing arrhythmia, as the success rate is poor. Medical therapy should be instituted in all patients with confirmed arrhythmia. Recent practice has advocated that first line treatment for AF should include cardioselective beta blockers, rate limiting calcium channel blockers and digoxin reserved for second line therapy. Amiodarone is principally used in older patients as it has no proven positive prognostic effects. It is an extremely useful antidysrhythmic but it has numerous side-effects of which the patient must be made aware. These include:

- Skin (slate grey pigmentation and photosensitivity)
- Pulmonary fibrosis (this is rare in doses below 400 mg per day)
- Thyroid dysfunction (it may cause both hyper- and hypothyroidism)
- Hepatitis.

It is important therefore to have baseline LFTs, TFTs and pulmonary function tests, and to record that the patient has been made aware of the possible side-effects.

Answer 9

(a) (i) Infective endocarditis *(1 mark)*

    (ii) Osler's nodes – painful, red indurating lesions in the finger pulps
Janeway lesions – macular, non-tender lesions on the palm and soles
Roth spots – retinal haemorrhages with pale, exudative centres *(3 marks)*

(b) Two to three sets of blood cultures before starting antibiotics
Echocardiogram *(2 marks)*

(c) Cardiovascular:
    Cardiac failure, pericarditis
    Aortic root abscess
    Haemolytic anaemia
Systemic:
    Meningitis, meningo-encephalitis
    Mycotic aneurysms
    Left-sided valves – systemic emboli
    Right-sided valves – pulmonary emboli
    Renal failure *(4 marks)*

Comment

Infective endocarditis may present in an acute or chronic manner, the acute form often running a malignant course. Although there are many people potentially at risk in the general population, the advent of antibiotics and the reduction in incidence of rheumatic valvular disease has meant the pattern and outcome of the disease has changed for the better over the 20th century. The disease is now more prevalent in men and is becoming increasingly prevalent in the elderly population. However, despite the improvements in prognosis, the acute form, particularly when caused by *Staphylococcus aureus* and *Streptococcus pneumoniae* infections, still carries a 30% mortality rate.

Common causative organisms include:

- *Streptococci* (*viridans, milleri, bovis, sanguis* and *mutans*)
- *Staphylococci* (*aureus, epidermidis, hominis*)
- Gram-negative organisms
- *Pseudomonas*
- HACEK group (*Haemophilus* spp, *Actinobacillus, Actinomyces comitans, Cardiobacterium hominis, Eikenella corrodens, Kingella kingae*)

Rarer organisms include *Coxiella burnetii, Brucella, Klebsiella* and *E. coli*. Any patient presenting with signs of sepsis and a cardiac murmur should alert the clinician to possible endocarditis. In the elderly it is always a diagnosis to exclude, as it often presents in a non-specific manner. Blood cultures are positive in 90%–95% of patients, and attempts should be made to obtain two to three sets in the hour before commencing antibiotic therapy. Echocardiography is the only other specific investigation, and is also quite sensitive. In patients for whom aortic root disease is suspected transoesophageal echo should be considered. Empirical treatment is often used in the severely sick or acute presentation, and consists of intravenous penicillin and gentamicin. If *Staphylococcus* is suspected then flucloxacillin may be added.

Answer 10

(a) Hypertrophic obstructive cardiomyopathy (HOCM)
Autosomal dominant   (*2 marks*)

(b) Ischaemic heart disease, hypertension, alcohol, sarcoidosis   (*3 marks*)

(c) Investigations:
Resting ECG; 48-hour tape
CXR
Echocardiogram with Doppler
Exercise testing with continuous BP monitoring
Medical therapy:
Amiodarone
Beta-blockers
Calcium-channel blockers
Surgical intervention:
Resection of outflow tract
In familial cases such as this, sibling and children
screening   *(5 marks)*

Comment

HOCM is an idiopathic disorder, which is usually familial, and is inherited in an autosomal dominant manner. Chromosomal analysis of families with the disease have identified abnormalities in the genes for troponin, myosin and tropomyosin. Clinically, patients present with symptoms of ventricular outflow tract obstruction or tachyarrhythmia. Chest pain, dyspnoea, palpitations and syncope are common, but there may be few symptoms prior to sudden death. Examination is often unremarkable, but may reveal signs of left or right ventricular outflow tract obstruction and associated dysfunction, which is commoner in younger patients. The classical murmur associated with HOCM is mid-systolic, and is accompanied by a forceful apex beat and a fourth heart sound. The intensity of the murmur is increased with exercise. Investigation is aimed at identifying the subgroup of patients with non-sustained ventricular tachycardia (VT), which has the greatest bearing on prognosis and, in particular, the likelihood of sudden death. Therefore essential investigations must include a 48-hour tape. Echocardiography with colour Doppler flow has recently superseded angiography in the younger patient. It can be used to assess not only the left ventricular dimensions and function but also the outflow tract. Cardiac catheter studies are now principally reserved for patients over the age of 40 to assess the coronary circulation. Specific therapy in those with non-sustained VT should include amiodarone. Propranolol and verapamil are also used. Patients with outflow tract gradients greater than 50 mmHg should be considered for surgical resection. Newer interventions including implantable defibrillator devices, pacemakers and alcohol ablation of the affected septum are also now commonly used.

Answer 11

(a) Fallot's tetralogy
Eisenmenger's syndrome (right to left shunt across a ventricular septal defect)
Transposition of the great vessels   *(3 marks)*

(b) Right ventricular outflow tract obstruction – usually pulmonary valvular stenosis
Ventricular septal defect, with an overriding aorta
Right ventricular hypertrophy   *(4 marks)*

(c) Surgical repair is the only curative treatment. It is usually divided into two procedures:
(i) palliative shunt formation, followed six months to one year later by
(ii) complete repair
In patients presenting with advanced disease – palliation with diuretics and oxygen   *(3 marks)*

Comment

Patients who undergo surgical correction for Fallot's tetralogy generally do very well, and go on to live normal lives. With advances in obstetric antenatal imaging and paediatric screening, most cases are picked up early and few now present with advanced disease. Initial surgical correction involves the formation of a palliative shunt between the pulmonary and systemic vasculature. This is particularly important when pulmonary atresia or severe polycythaemia is present. The aim of the shunt is to increase blood flow through the pulmonary vasculature and the left side of the heart. The shunts used are:

- Blalock (subclavian artery to either pulmonary artery)
- Waterston (ascending thoracic aorta to the right pulmonary artery)
- Potts (descending thoracic aorta to the left pulmonary artery)

Women who have had any congenital heart defect are at greater risk of having children with heart defects and therefore must be carefully monitored with foetal echocardiography throughout their pregnancy.

Answer 12

(a) Acute left ventricular failure – this is the most likely diagnosis
Tachyarrhythmia – atrial fibrillation, ventricular tachycardia or fibrillation
Reinfarction
Asthma
Bronchospasm secondary to β-blockade
Pulmonary embolism   *(3 marks)*

(b) FBC, U&Es, glucose, cardiac enzymes (CK and AST)
CXR
ECG
ABGs   *(3 marks)*

(c) Sit the patient upright
Oxygen via face mask
IV access
IV furosemide 40–80 mg ± IV diamorphine and anti-emetic
If severe consider IV nitrate infusion and urinary catheter
Monitor BP, pulse, oxygen saturation, cardiac monitor
If haemodynamically compromised – will need central venous line and inotrope support   *(4 marks)*

Comment

Left ventricular failure is a common complication of acute myocardial infarction. It may be precipitated by:

- Reinfarction or ongoing unstable angina
- Acute mitral regurgitation*
- Acute ventricular septal defect*

*Both may be inferred by a new pansystolic murmur

- Haemopericardium or acute ventricular rupture
- Arrhythmia (AF, SVT, VF or VT, complete heart block and bradyarrhythmia)
- Beta-blockade with existing impaired left ventricular function

Acute therapy is largely dependent on the haemodynamic status of the patient. If the patient is maintaining a reasonable blood pressure (>100 mmHg systolic) then IV loop diuretics and then IV nitrates should be employed which 'off load' the heart. Intravenous diamorphine may also be used. This acts as an anxiolytic, but also has local pulmonary effects. All of these treatments cause hypotension, and it is therefore important to monitor the patient at all times. Patients who are haemodynamically compromised should have a central venous line and urinary catheter inserted, to monitor fluid balance. They will also require inotrope support with dobutamine and in severe cases adrenaline and noradrenaline. Underlying factors, such as arrhythmia, need to be treated and mechanical problems, such as acute ventricular septal defect or mitral regurgitation, require surgical intervention.

Answer 13

(a) (i) Aortic stenosis *(1 mark)*
(ii) Congenital bicuspid valve
Rheumatic valvular disease *(2 marks)*

(b) Slow rising pulse
Narrow pulse pressure
Non-displaced heaving apex beat
Ejection systolic murmur, radiating to the carotids

(3 marks)

(c) Investigations:
CXR, ECG, echocardiogram, cardiac catheter studies
Management:
Aortic valve replacement (unless medically
contraindicated)

(4 marks)

Comment

Aortic stenosis is a common valvular disorder, primarily caused by degenerative change in a congenitally bicuspid valve. The commonest acquired cause remains rheumatic valvular disease. Clinically the patient presents with symptoms of left ventricular dysfunction and outflow tract obstruction. In significant disease this usually manifests itself as exertional angina, pulmonary oedema and exertional syncope. It may also cause sudden death.

Examination of the patient reveals a slow rising pulse with a low volume. The pulse pressure is narrow. The apex beat is non-displaced and is hyperdynamic or 'heaving' in nature. On auscultation there is an ejection systolic murmur which radiates to the carotids. The aortic component of the second heart sound may be soft or absent with reverse splitting of this sound. There may also be a fourth heart sound, and an ejection click. All patients require both echocardiography and cardiac catheter studies, the latter to assess both the gradient across the valve and the coronary circulation. Surgical replacement of the valve is the only curative treatment. Diuretic therapy maybe instituted in the inoperable or acute presentation, but should not be prolonged if surgery is being contemplated as it may exacerbate the condition.

Answer 14

(a) FBC, U&Es, glucose, lipids
Urinalysis – protein, blood, glucose
CXR
ECG   *(2 marks)*

(b) Diuretics – bendrofluazide
Beta-blockers – atenolol, oxprenolol
Calcium-channel blockers – diltiazem, verapamil,
nifedipine, amlodipine, lacidipine
ACEI – lisinopril, perindopril
Alpha-blockers – doxazosin
Angiotensin II antagonists – valsartan, candesartan,
irbesartan   *(4 marks)*

(c) Address all risk factors:
Smoking, alcohol excess, obesity, lack of exercise,
diabetes mellitus, hyperlipidaemia (these will need to
be reviewed by a dietician and specialist diabetic
liaison nurse)
Institute medical therapy – tailored to the individual
patient   *(4 marks)*

Comment

Essential or primary hypertension is responsible for 90%–95% of
all cases of hypertensive disease. It is a complex multifactorial
disorder, which arises due to interactions of genetic and
environmental factors. Several genes in combination predispose an
individual to develop hypertension, but it is exposure to various
environmental factors which determines expression and
progression of the disease. These factors include:

• **Diet** – various components of our diet have been related to the
development of hypertension. Excess sodium and low potassium
intake have both been postulated, but there remains limited
evidence to support this. Vegetarians have lower blood pressure
than their age-matched omnivorous counterparts, but this may
also be multifactorial

- **Obesity** – this involves neuroendocrine dysfunction and environmental factors such as lack of exercise
- **Alcohol excess** – greater than six units of alcohol per day is known to cause hypertension. Conversely, reduction in alcohol intake will lower the blood pressure
- **Environmental stress** – although this is known to cause acute rises in blood pressure, its long-term effects remain unknown
- **Lack of exercise** – improving exercise participation not only lowers blood pressure, it also improves prognosis in other related cardiovascular disease, eg biventricular cardiac failure

All of these risk factors, as well as diabetes and hyperlipidaemia, need to be addressed as medical therapy is being instituted.

With the wide range of antihypertensive agents available, therapy should now be tailored to an individual case. ACE inhibitors should be used in hypertensive diabetics as they retard onset of microvascular complications and have a slight positive effect on lipid profiles. Doxazosin, an α-adrenoceptor blocker, is particularly useful in resistant hypertension, where two to three agents in combination have failed to lower the blood pressure. It also has beneficial effects on the lipid profile and is therefore used in patients with associated hyperlipidaemia. In the older patient, bendrofluazide remains the first-line treatment, where the lower dose of 2.5 mg once a day (as compared to 5 mg) has been shown to be optimal.

See http://www.bhsoc.org/Other_Guidelines.stm

Answer 15

(a) Phaeochromocytoma
Cushing's syndrome
Conn's syndrome
Acromegaly   (3 marks)

(b) Renal artery stenosis
Polycystic kidney disease
Renal malignant tumours   *(3 marks)*

(c) Blood tests:
FBC, U&Es, glucose, calcium/phosphate, lipids
autoantibody screen, ANCA, ANF
Urine:
Dipstix for protein and glucose, microscopy for red
cell casts, consider 24-hour urine for protein and
creatinine clearance
Imaging:
Plain AXR, USS of kidneys, bladder, and ureters
consider IVU and renal DSA scan
This screen should indicate whether this is a renal or
extrarenal problem   *(4 marks)*

Comment

Secondary causes of hypertension are uncommon, accounting for
only 5% of cases. Of these, 80% are renal or renovascular in origin
and always need to be excluded in anyone presenting with
hypertension. Simple bedside tests including urine dipstix and
microscopy are often enough to exclude major renal disease. If
there is evidence of renal dysfunction on screening, then renal
imaging should be undertaken, including USS, IVP and DSA scan.
Other causes of chronic renal disease include the systemic
vasculitides, which should be excluded by an autoantibody screen,
in particular an ANCA test. The remaining 20% of cases are
principally associated with endocrine disorders.
Phaeochromocytoma, Cushing's syndrome, acromegaly, Conn's
syndrome and hyperparathyroidism may be excluded clinically,
biochemically, and by specific imaging and hormone assessment.

ANSWERS

Haematology

Answer 1

(a) Polycythaemia   *(1 mark)*

(b) Relative polycythaemia: with plasma volume contraction

Absolute polycythaemia: secondary to appropriate erythropoietin production, eg chronic carbon monoxide exposure.

secondary to exogenous erythropoietin abuse in athletes

secondary to inappropriate

erythropoietin production, eg in hepatocellular carcinoma, renal cell carcinoma, cerebellar haemangioblastoma or polycystic kidney disease erythropoietin-independent, eg polycythaemia vera or inherited activating mutations of the erythropoietin receptor

(4 marks)

(c) (i) Phlebotomy, aiming for haematocrit <45%, with low-dose aspirin except in patients at highest risk of haemorrhage. Hydroxyurea, interferon-alpha, anagrelide, imatinib mesylate and stem cell transplantation are sometimes used.

(ii) Survival of 10 years or more is usual. Morbidity and mortality occur as a result of thrombosis, major haemorrhage or transformation to acute leukaemia or 'spent phase' myelofibrosis.

(5 marks)

Comment

Red blood cell production is primarily regulated by erythropoietin, a hormone secreted by peritubular interstitial cells in the kidney, in response to reduced tissue oxygen tension. Polycythaemia, an abnormal increase in haematocrit, may thus arise from a relative reduction in plasma volume, from an increase in circulating erythropoietin concentration, or from an erythropoietin-independent expansion of erythroid precursors in the bone marrow.

Answer 2

(a) Factor IX
Prothrombin complex concentrate (factors II, VII, IX and X)
Activated prothrombin complex concentrate (factors IIa, VIIa, IXa and Xa)
Fresh-frozen plasma
Factor VIIa   *(4 marks)*

(b) Genetic mutation in factor IX gene
Leads to a deficiency of factor IX
Causes inability to form tenase complex allowing activation of factor X   *(3 marks)*

(c)   Acute thrombosis
      Development of inhibitor antibodies
      Anaphylaxis
      Transfusion-related viral infection (HIV, hepatitis B, C,
      D, G, parvovirus B19)
      Liver cirrhosis, liver failure or hepatocellular carcinoma
      secondary to chronic viral hepatitis
      Transfusion-related prion infection (CJD, vCJD)
                                                    (3 marks)

Comment

Haemophilia B is caused by a chromosome X-linked genetic
deficiency in clotting factor IX. The clinical features are similar to
those of haemophilia A (factor VIII deficiency), with the most
severely affected patients suffering spontaneous haemorrhage into:

- Joints (haemarthrosis), causing debilitating arthropathy
- Central nervous system, causing neurological disability
- Soft tissues, causing compartment syndrome, peripheral nerve
  compression and, occasionally, acute hypovolaemia

In the setting of an acute bleed, or for prophylaxis during surgery,
intravenous administration of recombinant factor IX restores
clotting ability. Recombinant factor VIIa is an alternative for
patients who have formed inhibitory antibodies against factor IX,
which, to them, is a foreign antigen. When specialist clotting factor
products are not immediately available, fresh-frozen plasma is a
useful stopgap treatment for life-threatening haemorrhage.
Cryoprecipitate contains factor VIII but not factor IX, so is useful
for emergency treatment of haemophilia A but not haemophilia B.

Prior to the introduction of donor screening, concentrate
purification techniques and recombinant factor preparations,
transmission of viruses in contaminated clotting factor
concentrates resulted in many haemophilia sufferers contracting
HIV and the hepatitis viruses. More recently, the possibility of
transmission of infectious prions has caused much concern.

Answer 3

(a) Clinical: Back pain
                     Tachycardia
                     Hypotension
                     Dyspnoea
                     Fever
                     Rigors
    Laboratory: Elevated serum bilirubin (unconjugated)
                     Elevated serum lactate dehydrogenase
                     Urinalysis haemoglobin positive
                     Direct antigen test (Coomb's test)
                     positive   *(4 marks)*

(b) ABO incompatibility   *(1 mark)*

(c) Stop the transfusion immediately
    Treat as medical emergency
    High-flow oxygen
    ECG monitoring
    Move to high dependency environment
    Intravenous 0.9% (normal) saline diuresis
    Withdraw fresh cross-match sample and send to
    laboratory with suspect unit of blood
    Endotracheal intubation, ventilation, inotropic
    support and haemofiltration or dialysis may be
    necessary   *(5 marks)*

Comment

Acute haemolytic transfusion reactions occur when antibodies in the recipient's blood react against antigen on the surface of transfused red blood cells. Complement activation and haemolysis occur, followed rapidly by the release of inflammatory cytokines, which may lead to circulatory collapse. The commonest reason for transfusion of an incompatible unit is misidentification of the patient, either at the time of phlebotomy or of setting up the transfusion.

The clinical features of an acute haemolytic transfusion reaction may begin after transfusion of just 5–10 ml of incompatible blood. Back pain is usual, and is accompanied by dyspnoea, hypotension, tachycardia, fever, rigors and diaphoresis. Renal failure may occur as a result of hypotension and haemoglobin deposition. These processes may be ameliorated by encouraging diuresis with intravenous crystalloids.

Other causes of severe acute transfusion reaction include infusion of bacterially contaminated blood products, anaphylaxis, and transfusion-related acute lung injury. In contrast to acute haemolytic and other severe transfusion reactions, febrile non-haemolytic transfusion reactions are very common. Since they usually result from interaction between recipient antibody and donor white cells and platelets, their incidence is decreased by measures that reduce the number of white cells in transfused blood components. They may also be prevented by premedication with paracetamol or a glucocorticoid.

Answer 4

(a) Acute autoimmune cold haemagglutinin disease secondary to *Mycoplasma pneumoniae* infection

(2 marks)

(b) (i) Polychromasia (anisochromia)
Macrocytosis
Reticulocytosis
Poikilocytosis

(ii) Direct Coombs' (antiglobulin) test – positive
Plasma haptoglobin – reduced
Serum bilirubin (unconjugated) – elevated
Serum lactate dehydrogenase – elevated
Urine urobilinogen – elevated   *(3 marks)*

(c) Inherited:

Membrane defects, eg hereditary spherocytosis

Metabolic defects, eg glucose-6-phosphate deficiency

Haemoglobin defects, eg sickle cell disease

Acquired:

Autoimmune, eg warm and cold haemolytic anaemias

Isoimmune, eg haemolytic transfusion reactions, haemolytic disease of the newborn

Non-immune, eg prosthetic valves, malaria, drug reactions *(5 marks)*

Comment

Normal red blood cells survive for approximately 120 days. If haemolysis occurs, healthy bone marrow with an adequate haematinic supply can maintain a normal haematocrit until the cell life span is reduced to about 15 days. Anaemia is inevitable beyond this point.

Extravascular haemolysis involves phagocytosis by macrophages in the spleen, liver, bone marrow and other components of the reticuloendothelial system. Splenic enlargement is typical, and splenomegaly is sometimes indicated to reduce the rate of haemolysis. Extravascular haemolysis occurs in:

- Inherited haemolytic anaemias, eg hereditary spherocytosis, thalassaemias
- Chronic drug reactions, eg to methyldopa, mefenamic acid
- Chronic immune processes, eg warm autoimmune haemolytic anaemia

Intravascular haemolysis typically occurs in acute conditions and may cause renal failure as well as anaemia. Haemoglobin released directly into the plasma during intravascular haemolysis binds to haptoglobin, a transport protein synthesised by the liver. Haemoglobin–haptoglobin complexes are removed from the circulation by the reticuloendothelial system. The serum haptoglobin level is thus a sensitive marker of intravascular haemolysis. Unbound free haemoglobin degrades in the circulation, resulting in unconjugated bilirubinaemia, methaemalbuminaemia (causing brown discoloration of the plasma) and elevated faecal and urinary urobilinogen levels. It is also filtered in the kidneys, resulting in haemosiderin deposition in the renal tubules, with subsequent shedding of affected cells, and in haemoglobinuria. Acute renal failure follows in the most severe cases. Intravascular haemolysis occurs in:

- Direct red cell trauma, eg microangiopathic haemolytic anaemia, turbulent flow around damaged metallic cardiac valve prostheses
- Complement-mediated attack, eg cold haemagglutinin disease, acute haemolytic transfusion reactions
- Other acute haemolytic crises, eg fulminant *Plasmodium falciparum* malaria (blackwater fever) or acute drug, infection and fava bean reactions in inherited glucose-6-phosphate deficiency

Answer 5

(a) Iron-deficiency anaemia
Anaemia of chronic disease
Thalassaemia trait
Sideroblastic anaemia – primary and secondary
(3 marks)

(b) FBC, with MCV, MCH and MCHC
Iron studies – iron, TIBC
Ferritin
Haemoglobin electrophoresis – in suspected thalassaemia
Consider bone marrow examination
Upper and lower gastrointestinal endoscopy or barium studies
Cervical smear and pelvic USS   *(3 marks)*

(c) Gastrointestinal:

Upper: oesophagitis, oesophageal carcinoma,
varices, hiatus hernia
peptic ulcer disease
benign tumours of the stomach,
eg leiomyoma
malignant tumours of the stomach

Lower: anal fissures, haemorrhoids, rectal ulcer,
rectal carcinoma
diverticular disease, inflammatory bowel
disease, colonic carcinoma, infective colitis,
angiodysplasia

Extra-intestinal:

Gynaecological:
fibroids, dysfunctional uterine bleeding
menorrhagia – primary and secondary,
cervical and uterine carcinoma

Epistaxis

Urinary tract:
renal tumours, polycystic kidneys
bladder tumours   *(4 marks)*

Comment

Anaemia is a clinical sign and wherever possible needs a definitive underlying diagnosis. Microcytic anaemia is principally caused by iron deficiency, but may also be caused by anaemia of chronic disease, thalassaemia trait and sideroblastic anaemia.

Iron-deficiency anaemia is characterised by a hypochromic, microcytic picture and is most commonly caused by blood loss. It is associated with a low ferritin and low plasma iron. The commonest cause worldwide is infestation of the gut by hookworm. In the Western world, menstrual loss is the commonest cause, but in all cases gastrointestinal pathology should be excluded. Particularly in male patients over the age of 40 and postmenopausal women, malignancy must be excluded, and upper and lower gastrointestinal investigation with endoscopy or barium studies are mandatory. Anaemia of chronic disease arises secondary to chronic inflammatory disorders, such as inflammatory bowel disease or rheumatological conditions, and is associated with a moderate reduction of the MCV, and normal iron and ferritin levels. Alpha- and β-thalassaemia trait are identifiable by a disproportionate reduction in the MCV compared to the minor level of anaemia, eg Hb 10.5 g/dl, MCV 63 fl (normal range 80–96 fl). They can be confirmed by haemoglobin electrophoresis. The sideroblastic anaemias are relatively uncommon. They may be congenital, due to a rare X-linked enzyme defect in the haem synthesis pathway, or acquired, secondary to malignancy, myeloproliferative disorders and toxins, such as alcohol and lead. Often, however, no cause is found. They are characterised by ring sideroblasts in the bone marrow.

Answer 6

(a) Hypothyroidism
   Pernicious anaemia/vitamin B12 deficiency   *(2 marks)*

(b) Pernicious anaemia is caused by one of two antibodies directed against intrinsic factor (IF), thus blocking vitamin B12 absorption
   Type I – blocks the binding of intrinsic factor to vitamin B12
   Type II – blocks the IF: vitamin B12 complex binding to its receptor site in the terminal ileum   *(3 marks)*

(c) Investigations:
   FBC, U&Es, TFTs, glucose
   Vitamin B12/folate
   Autoimmune antibody screen
   Treatment:
   Thyroxine replacement
   Vitamin B12 injections every three months
   This woman should also have an upper gastrointestinal endoscopy to exclude carcinoma of the stomach, which occurs in 2% of cases   *(5 marks)*

Comment

Macrocytosis, ie an MCV > 96 fl, may be classified according to the presence or absence of megaloblasts in the peripheral blood film. When associated with megaloblasts, vitamin B12 and folate deficiencies are the commonest causes. These are both classically associated with hypersegmented neutrophils. Macrocytosis in the absence of megaloblastic changes may occur physiologically in the newborn and pregnancy, and is pathologically associated with chronic liver disease, alcohol abuse, hypothyroidism and reticulocytosis. Pernicious anaemia is an autoimmune disorder predominantly occurring in older women. It is commonly associated with other autoimmune disorders, including hypothyroidism, vitiligo and Addison's disease. Autoantibodies directed against intrinsic factor and the terminal ileal binding sites stop vitamin B12 absorption, leading to a macrocytic anaemia. Treatment of the anaemia is by intramuscular vitamin B12 injection. Initially, five 1-mg loading injections are given over two weeks, and then maintenance doses are subsequently given every three months.

Answer 7

(a) (i) Alpha- and beta-thalassaemia
Hb SC disease
Hb D and Hb E disease *(2 marks)*
(ii) Acute splenic sequestration *(1 mark)*

(b) Treat the underlying cause of the acute sickle crisis
IV access, IV fluids to maintain adequate hydration
Oxygen via mask
Appropriate analgesia – opiates
Blood transfusion if required *(3 marks)*

(c) (i) Skin – chronic leg ulceration
(ii) Renal – acute and chronic papillary necrosis
(iii) Biliary tree – pigmented gallstones
(iv) Bone – aseptic necrosis of the femoral head
(4 marks)

Comment

Haemolytic anaemias are characterised by features of:

- Increased red cell production (reticulocytosis)
- Increased red cell destruction (unconjugated hyperbilirubinaemia)
- Red cell damage (fragmentation and shortened red cell survival)

The haemoglobinopathies are caused by defective globin chain synthesis and all result in haemolysis of varying severity. The thalassaemias are caused by absent or abnormal production of the alpha (α) and beta (β) chains which form the normal adult haemoglobin, Hb A, ($\alpha2\beta2$). The clinically significant haemoglobinopathies are summarised below.

Alpha-thalassaemia

αo – homozygous – no α chain production, is incompatible with life and causes the death of the foetus, termed hydrops fetalis. The resulting Hb is called Hb Barts, and has four gamma chains.

α+ – heterozygotes – there is some α chain production allowing normal Hb A and Hb $\beta4$ to be produced. This gives rise to mild to moderate haemolytic disease.

Beta-thalassaemia

βo – homozygotes – severe haemolytic disease, requiring repeated transfusion.

β+ – heterozygotes – usually symptomless.

$\delta\beta$ – mild to moderate disease, due to the depletion of δ chain gene. The δ chain forms part of the Hb A2, which accounts for 2% of adult haemoglobin

Sickle cell disease (Hb S)

Hb SS – homozygotes – this is a common haemoglobinopathy in Black races and is caused by an amino acid abnormality at position 6 of the β chain. It presents in acute sickle 'crises', usually precipitated by infection. The various organs involved are damaged through micro-infarcts, which lead to the bony pain, renal failure and chronic skin ulceration.

Heterozygotes usually remain symptomless until exposed to a stress, such as hypoxia or major surgery.

Hb S may combine with other Hb defects, eg Hb S/β-thalassaemia, and Hb SC disease.

The other chain defects give rise to:

- Hb C disease (this is a β chain abnormality principally found in West Africa)
- Hb D disease (mild haemolytic disease)
- Hb E disease (this occurs mainly in South East Asia and produces a mild haemolytic disease)

The persistence of these genetic defects is associated with protection against malarial infection.

Answer 8

(a) Lymphoma – probably Hodgkin's disease   *(1 mark)*

(b) FBC and blood film, ESR
CXR
Lymph node biopsy
Bone marrow trephine
Staging CT scan of the thorax and abdomen   *(5 marks)*

(c) Therapeutic management depends on the stage of the disease at presentation:
Radiotherapy – palliative or curative
Chemotherapy – combination therapy given in cycles
Autologous bone marrow transplant – given with total body irradiation or chemotherapy   *(4 marks)*

Comment

Lymphomas are divided into Hodgkin's and non-Hodgkin's disease. Hodgkin's disease has a bimodal age presentation, the early peak at 20 to 30 years, and the later peak over the age of 50. It is twice as common in men. The diagnosis is confirmed by histology from biopsied lymph nodes, and is characterised by the presence of the Reed–Sternberg cell. The histology also defines the classification and prognosis, as shown below.

Histological variety	Survival at five years (%)
Lymphocyte predominant	80–85
Nodular sclerosing	80
Mixed cellularity	60
Lymphocyte depleted	50

Each stage is subdivided into a and b, depending on the absence or presence of systemic symptoms, respectively, eg night sweats and pruritus.

The non-Hodgkin's lymphomas are a relatively heterogeneous group, with variable presentations and progression. They are classified by their malignant potential into low-, intermediate- and high-grade lymphomas, and by their cell type into T-cell and B-cell diseases. Certain diseases predispose to this group of malignancies, including immunosuppressive disorders, eg AIDS, EBV, coeliac disease, rheumatoid arthritis and SLE. The prognosis varies from 80%–90% survival at five years in low-grade disease, to 40%–50% survival in high-grade disease.

Answer 9

(a) Viral respiratory tract infection, leading to immune thrombocytopenic purpura *(2 marks)*

(b) Aplastic anaemia – idiopathic (50%), drugs, sepsis
Hypersplenism, eg chronic haemolytic disease
Myelofibrosis
DIC
SLE *(5 marks)*

(c)   Usually self-limiting – can have spontaneous
      remissions
      Steroids are used in more severe cases
      In chronic disease – splenectomy or
      immunosuppressants   *(3 marks)*

Comment

Reduced platelet numbers or thrombocytopenia is characterised
by purpura, easy bruising and overt bleeding, such as
menorrhagia, epistaxis and gastrointestinal bleeds. Treatment in
severe cases requires blood transfusion, FFP and platelets,
although if the underlying cause is not corrected, giving platelets
has little effect. In chronic thrombocytopenia treatment is
principally steroids and immunosuppressants, such as
azathioprine, cyclophosphamide and chlorambucil.

Thrombocytopenia may be classified into reduced platelet
production or increased destruction as shown below:

- Reduced production (congenital)
- Reduced production (acquired – marrow infiltration,
  eg myelofibrosis, aplastic anaemia, drugs, eg omeprazole,
  megaloblastosis)
- Increased destruction (immune – idiopathic, viral, drugs)
- Increased destruction (microangiopathic disease – TTP, DIC,
  HUS)
- Increased destruction (septicaemia – usually secondary to
  Gram-negative organisms)

Answer 10

(a)   Acute lymphoblastic leukaemia (ALL)
      It has a higher incidence in association with trisomy 21
                                                   (2 marks)

(b) FBC with blood film
CXR
Bone marrow aspirate and trephine
Lymph node biopsy
Chromosome analysis
Cytochemistry and immune markers   *(3 marks)*

(c) General supportive treatment:
    Nutritional support, blood transfusions
    Neutropenic patients – isolated, infection
Prophylaxis and treatment
Specific cytotoxic therapy
Radiotherapy
Maintenance therapy
Relapse treatment – bone marrow transplant and
chemotherapy   *(5 marks)*

Comment

Acute lymphoblastic (ALL) and acute myeloid (AML) leukaemia present most commonly with symptoms of bone marrow failure, ie anaemia, recurrent infection, easy bruising and overt bleeding.

ALL presents in childhood, with bone marrow failure, hepatosplenomegaly and lymphadenopathy. Other less common sites of primary infiltration are the gums, skin, thyroid, central nervous system and testes, although these are often sites of recurrence.

The incidence of AML increases with age, and presents similarly to ALL, often with associated systemic symptoms such as malaise, fever and lethargy. The acute leukaemias are classified by cell morphology, immunological markers and cytochemical staining. The main classification is the FAB, ie French, American and British.

Prognosis is now estimated at 60% at five years for ALL, but spontaneous relapses, resistance and complications to the initial treatment will significantly reduce this.

Poor prognostic indicators at presentation include:

- WCC > 20·10⁹/l
- Male
- Presenting age < 2 and > 10 years
- B-ALL
- Philadelphia chromosome or other translocations
- Central nervous system involvement
- Slow remission

Answer 11

(a) (i) Chronic myeloid leukaemia (CML)   *(1 mark)*
   (ii) Philadelphia chromosome. This is a reciprocal
      translocation between chromosomes 9 and 22
                                                   (1 mark)

(b) Chronic malaria
   Visceral leishmaniasis
   Myelofibrosis
   Gaucher's disease   *(2 marks)*

(c) (i) FBC and blood film
      Chromosome analysis
      Neutrophil alkaline phosphatase score
      Bone marrow aspirate and trephine   *(3 marks)*
   (ii) Treatment:
        Cytotoxic therapy
        Imatinib
        Bone marrow transplant
        Splenic irradiation or splenectomy
        Allopurinol   *(3 marks)*

Comment

The chronic-myeloid and lymphocytic leukaemias (CML and
CLL) present in middle and later life, although they may rarely
occur in children. CML has a peak presentation between 40 and 60
years of age, and presents with symptoms of bone marrow failure,
splenomegaly and systemic upset, such as malaise and fever. It is

characterised by the presence of the Philadelphia chromosome. Death occurs usually as the result of acute transformation, with secondary infection and severe marrow dysfunction. The prognosis for Philadelphia chromosome-positive CML sufferers has improved markedly since the introduction of imatinib (Glivec-Novartis), a protein-tyrosine kinase inhibitor that specifically targets the Bcr-abl gene.

CLL is usually a disorder of the elderly adult, being rare before the age of 40. It is often asymptomatic and picked up only on routine blood tests. It is classified according to the Rai staging system, as shown below:

- STAGE 0 (peripheral lymphocytosis >15 000/mm³/marrow lymphocytosis > 40%)
- STAGE 1 (stage 0 + lymphadenopathy)
- STAGE 2 (stage 1 + splenomegaly and/or hepatomegaly)
- STAGE 3 (stage 2 + Hb < 11 g/dl)
- STAGE 4 (stage 3 + platelet count < 100 000/mm³)

Older, asymptomatic patients often require no specific treatment, but in more advanced cases, particularly in patients with stage 3 or 4 disease, general support (ie nutritional and psychological support), early treatment of infection, and chemotherapy, radiotherapy and splenectomy are all employed. The median survival is 12 to 15 years in stage 0 disease, and one to three years in stage 4 disease.

Answer 12

(a) Pathological fracture
Multiple myeloma   *(2 marks)*

(b) FBC and blood film
U&Es
Calcium and phosphate
ESR
Plasma electrophoresis
Urinary Bence Jones proteins
Bone marrow aspirate   *(5 marks)*

(c)   IV access
      IV fluids – rehydrate using normal saline
      Principal treatment:
         IV bisphosphanates, eg pamidronate
         Consider loop diuretics, steroids and calcitonin

(3 marks)

Comment

Multiple myeloma is a malignant condition of the bone marrow,
which presents after the age of 40. It is characterised by the
presence of plasma cells in the marrow, lytic bone lesions and a
monoclonal paraprotein, which is found in the plasma and urine.
This paraprotein is most commonly IgG, followed by IgA and IgM.
IgD and combination cases are rare.

Clinically it presents with:

- Bony pain (particularly of the lower back)
- Features of bone marrow failure (anaemia, recurrent infection
  and overt bleeding)
- Hypercalcaemia (this produces nausea and vomiting, confusion,
  polyuria and polydipsia)
- Renal failure (renal impairment may be due to one of several
  mechanisms, deposition of light chains in the tubules,
  hypercalcaemia, hyperuricaemia, amyloidosis, pyelonephritis)

Treatment options have increased recently with significant
improvements in prognosis. Drugs such as thalidomide and
bortezomib are more effective than traditional alkylating agents
such as melphalan. Stem cell transplantation is possible for some
patients. Poor prognostic indicators at the time of presentation
include: severe anaemia, uraemia >14 mmol/l, high levels of Bence
Jones proteins, raised β2-microglobulin and a low albumin.

Dermatology

Answer 1

(a) Obstructive jaundice – probably secondary to
gallstones   *(1 mark)*

(b) Scabies
Eczema/dermatitis
Parasitic infestation
Iron-deficiency anaemia   *(4 marks)*

(c) Keep the patient cool
Keep skin well oiled with emollients
Avoid excessive bathing – drying
Treat the underlying disorder
Antihistamines
Sedatives
Low-dose amitriptyline (nocte)
Short nails
May require occlusive bandaging of skin   *(5 marks)*

Comment

Pruritus is a common symptom of many dermatoses and systemic
disorders. The sensation is produced in the skin by various
stimulants, such as bradykinins, histamine, proteases and bile salts,
and is relayed to the thalamus and sensory cortex via the lateral
spinothalamic tract. There are a number of important causes of
pruritus, which should always be excluded in any presentation. The
commonest in the UK include insect bites and scabies, where the
burrows and tracts should be sought in the skin webs of the fingers
and toes. Generalised pruritus accompanies several systemic
disorders. Biliary disease, particularly obstructive jaundice, presents

with pruritus caused by bile salt accumulation in the skin. Haematological disorders, including iron deficiency anaemia, CLL and Hodgkin's disease. Chronic uraemia classically due to PRV, chronic glomerulonephritis or chronic pyelonephritis may present with intense itching, which may be unrelieved, even with dialysis. Psychological factors such as depression may decrease the threshold of pruritus. Treatment should be aimed at the underlying condition if one is readily identifiable. Symptomatic relief should include night sedation, keeping the skin well oiled with emollients, with the patient cooled. Drug therapy may include low-dose amitriptyline and antihistamines. In haematological and biliary disease, a combination of H1 and H2 antagonists seem to produce a better response.

Answer 2

(a) (i)   Contact dermatitis   *(2 marks)*
     (ii) Nickel sensitivity – earrings, shampoos   *(1 mark)*

(b) Nickel fasteners on bras
     Metal buttons on clothes, jeans, shoes
     Rubber in the elastic of underwear
     Cosmetics and perfumes   *(3 marks)*

(c) Avoidance of sensitisers
     Should be recommended to wear gloves if continuing
     in her job
     Patch testing to confirm allergens
     Acute – steroid creams reduces inflammation
                                                                    (4 marks)

Comment

Contact dermatitis may be due to over-exposure to a particular irritant such as bleach, shampoo and cleaning agents, or may be an allergic phenomenon due to exposure to a sensitiser. Common sensitisers include cosmetics, particularly the cheaper varieties, nickel and metallic elements in clothing and shoes and plants. There are several occupation-related contact dermatoses, including hairdressers (nickel), farmers (pesticides) and builders (chrome). Treatment is based on identification of a sensitising allergen, and then avoidance if possible. Acutely, anti-inflammatory agents may be needed, steroid creams being most useful. Stress and the wellbeing of the patients are also very important in how the disorder is perceived and in the prognosis.

Answer 3

(a) Lichenification – thickening of the skin with increase of the skin markings due to excessive scratching and rubbing
Flexures of the limbs and creases of the face and neck
(3 marks)

(b) Atopic/extrinsic asthma
Allergic rhinitis
IgE-mediated response – associated with depressed T-cell response *(3 marks)*

(c) Acute treatment:
Moisturisation of the affected skin
Wet dressings with overlying dry dressing
Treatment of infected areas – IV antibiotics
Avoid drying agents/irritants – soaps
Steroid creams
Prevention:
Allergen avoidance – house dust mites
Irritant avoidance – soap, wool
Keep skin moisturised with emollients
'Short sharp bursts' of steroid creams
(4 marks)

Comment

Atopic eczema is a multifactorial allergic disorder affecting the skin, with 30%–50% of patients having associated atopic asthma or hayfever. Classically it presents three to six months postnatally, and by three years characteristically affects the flexures of the limbs and creases of the face and the neck.

The pathogenesis is based on a depressed T-cell response to environmental challenges, with an associated lack of suppression

of humoral immunity, principally IgE related. The allergens
involved are a heterogeneous group, including food substances,
house dust mites and pollens. The skin becomes reddened, dry and
intensely itchy, and subsequent scratching and rubbing lead to
breaking of the epidermis, ulceration and infection. Chronically
this leads to lichenification. Most patients 'grow out' of their atopy
by their early teenage years, and in the absence of major irritants,
their skin may return to normal. More severe cases may require
systemic as well as topical steroids. Other treatments include
topical calcineurin inhibitors (e.g. tacrolimus and pimecrolimus);
UV phototherapy and suptemic immunosuppressants such as
azathioprine and mycophenolate mofetil.

Answer 4

(a) Koebner phenomenon – the rash develops in a line
caused by the trauma of scratching
Lichen planus; discoid lupus erythematosus; vitiligo;
warts; eczema; secondary syphilis   *(3 marks)*

(b) Scalp; buttocks; truncal area
Nails
Joints   *(3 marks)*

(c) Topical:
corticosteroids – skin atrophy
vitamin D analogues – local irritation (common)
coal tar preparations – local irritation (rare)
dithranol paste – local irritation, particularly
genitalia and eyes
Systemic:
UV phototherapy – late skin cancers
corticosteroids – Cushing's syndrome
immunosuppressants, e.g. methotrexate –
opportunistic infections
anti-TNFa biological agents, e.g. etanercept – late
cancers
anti-T-cell biological agents, e.g. efalizumab –
opportunistic infections   *(4 marks)*

Comment

Psoriasis is a common dermatological disorder, which affects approximately 2% of the White population in the UK. It is less common in dark skinned races. It affects all age groups with a peak incidence in young adults. It is now known there are two modes of inheritance: type I, which is associated with HLA-CW6, -B13 and BW57 and has a strong family history; type II, which is the more common and is associated with HLA-CW2 and -B27. Pathologically it is characterised by an increase in the rate of epidermal cell turnover. Clinically there is epidermal thickening and scaling which most commonly occur in demarcated plaques. Psoriasis may occur in several patterns:

- Guttate – this is a 'droplet' type pattern which follows a streptococcal infection. It is common in children
- Pustular psoriasis – in this disorder pustules occur associated with a systemic upset, including pyrexia, arthropathy and erythema. It usually occurs in association with psoriatic treatment including steroids but, rarely, may be associated with hypothyroidism
- Nummular discoid – this is the commonest form associated with well demarcated plaques over the extensor surfaces

Answer 5

(a) Erythema multiforme, Stevens–Johnson syndrome

(2 marks)

(b) *Mycoplasma pneumonia*
Herpes simplex, *Streptococcus*, Orf virus
Drugs, eg penicillin, sulphonamides   *(4 marks)*

(c) Investigations:
        FBC, U&Es, LFTS
        Atypical pneumonia screen: *Mycoplasma, Legionella, Chlamydia*
        CXR, ABGs
     Treatment:
        Treat the underlying cause – amoxicillin and erythromycin
        Systemic steroids
        Nutrition must be addressed if prolonged mouth ulceration stops oral intake   *(4 marks)*

Comment

Erythema multiforme is characterised by the target lesion, which is a red annular lesion with a blistering centre. The rash predominantly affects the peripheries, but may also involve the trunk, genitalia, eyes and mouth. Common causes include:

- Bacteria (streptococcus, mycoplasma)
- Viruses (HSV, Orf)
- Fungi (histoplasmosis, coccidioidomycosis)
- Drugs (penicillins, sulphonamides, NSAIDs)
- Inflammatory bowel disease
- Rheumatoid arthritis and SLE
- Neoplasia
- Radiotherapy and chemotherapy

The Stevens–Johnson syndrome is a severe form of the more common erythema multiforme, presenting with blistering and mucosal involvement. It may be associated with multi-organ failure, and requires immediate attention. Treatment is based on symptomatic relief and treatment of the underlying disorder. The more severe Stevens–Johnson syndrome requires systemic steroids.

Answer 6

(a) Erythema nodosum *(1 mark)*

(b) Infection – TB
Drugs – sulphonamides
Inflammatory bowel disease (IBD)
Sarcoidosis *(4 marks)*

(c) Stop oral contraceptive pill (OCP); use other forms of
contraception
Analgesia with aspirin; bedrest
Treat underlying infection if present
Steroids – if not settling *(5 marks)*

Comment

Erythema nodosum is characterised by painful, tender, red lesions,
which are often ill-defined and merge into one another. They
occur over the anterior aspect of the shins, the forearms and more
rarely the truncal area.

Common causes include:

- Infection (bacterial: streptococcal, TB, lymphogranuloma
venereum, leprosy; viral: EBV; fungal: histoplasmosis,
blastomycosis, coccidioidomycosis)
- Sarcoidosis
- IBD
- Drugs (sulphonamides, OCP, bromides)
- Pregnancy
- Malignancy (leukaemia, lymphoma)

Management is based on treating the underlying cause. A chest
X-ray is mandatory as sarcoidosis and tuberculosis are common
associations. The rash is self-limiting but aspirin and bedrest are
recommended. Steroids may help with swelling and fever, but do
not change the duration of the illness. They may also be indicated
for treatment of the underlying disorder.

Answer 7

(a)   Pemphigus vulgaris, pemphigoid, fixed drug eruption, insect bites   *(3 marks)*

(b)   Do you have any ulcers/blisters in the mouth?
Have you started any new medications recently?
Have you been in contact with any biting insects recently, eg mites or mosquitoes?   *(3 marks)*

(c) (i)   Nikolsky's sign – sliding pressure applied to the edge of a lesion will cause the epidermis to break away
Diagnosis – Pemphigus vulgaris   *(2 marks)*

    (ii) Corticosteroids
Immunosuppressants, e.g. azathioprine, cyclophosphamide
Intravenous immunoglobulin (IVIG)
Rituximab   *(2 marks)*

Comment

Pemphigus is an autoimmune disorder caused by an antibody to desmogleins 1 and 3 within the epidermis. It is associated with HLA-A10 and -DR4, and is more common in Jews and in the Indian subcontinent. Clinically it presents with superficial blistering/erosive lesions, with a predilection for the buccal mucosa. The lesions classically exhibit Nikolsky's sign. Treatment is based on immunosuppression with high-dose corticosteroids, steroid-sparing agents and intravenous immunoglobulin. Rituximab, a therapeutic antibody that targets CD20 on B-cells, is used in refractory cases. Most patients are cured and therapy is usually stopped within two years.

Pemphigoid is a more common disorder than pemphigus, and presents with large, tense, bullous eruptions, principally in the over 60s population. It is unusual for it to affect the mouth. It is also an immune-mediated disorder and in 70% of cases there is a specific IgG targeted against the basement membrane of the epidermis. The treatment is similar to pemphigus, with most patients cured within one year.

Answer 8

(a) Rapid increasing size
Itching
Bleeding – spontaneous
Irregular margins
Development of any new pigmented lesion after
puberty
Associated surrounding lesions
Distant similar lesions
Recent change in surface
Change in colour
Lymph node enlargement   *(4 marks)*

(b) Basal cell carcinoma, squamous cell carcinoma, solar
keratoses, malignant melanoma, Bowen's disease
                                            (3 marks)

(c) Excision of naevus
Chemotherapy for metastatic disease
Advice about sunlight avoidance   *(3 marks)*

Comment

The incidence of malignant melanoma is rapidly increasing within
White populations, particularly in the UK. This is thought to be
principally due to Celtic, 'red haired' races, subjecting themselves to
short sharp bursts of intense sunbathing on summer holidays. The
most important prognostic indicator is the depth of the lesion
(known as the Breslow thickness):

- < 0.76 mm   (95% survival/5 years)
- > 0.76–1 mm   (80% survival/5 years)
- > 3.5 mm   (40% survival/5 years)

Recent studies have shown that wide excision with regional lymph
node dissection has no advantage over less radical surgery, and
presently the recommendation is 1 cm excision margins for every
1 mm in depth to a maximum of 3 cm. Trials continue with
various forms of chemotherapy, immunotherapy and vaccines.

Prophylaxis with ongoing education about the importance of 'covering up' in the sun, and the use of sun-screening agents, has been shown to be a successful influence in Australasia and southern Africa.

Answer 9

   (a)   Thyrotoxicosis
        Psoriasis   *(2 marks)*

   (b)   TFTs
        Nail clippings/scraping – UV (Wood's light)
        Thyroid autoantibodies
        HLA (1327) – karyotyping   *(2 marks)*

   (c)   (i)   Koilonychia
        (ii)   Clubbing
        (iii) Splinter haemorrhages and clubbing
        (iv) Pitting, transverse ridging, dystrophy, onycholysis
        (v)   Beau's lines
        (vi) Leukonychia, clubbing   *(6 marks)*

Comment

The nails of the digits continue to grow throughout life. Retardation in growth may occur in severe psychiatric or systemic disease; acceleration of nail growth occurs principally in psoriasis.

The shape of the nails varies in numerous systemic disorders.

Clubbing of the nail
Classically this is an increase in the curvature of the nail in both longitudinal and transverse planes, with loss of the angle between the nail bed and skin fold. The nail bed becomes fluctuant. Causes include:

- Idiopathic
- Chronic suppurative lung disease (CF, bronchiectasis, empyema, TB, abscess)
- Pulmonary malignancy

- Congenital cyanotic heart disease
- Infective endocarditis
- Inflammatory bowel disease
- Chronic liver disease
- Biliary disease

Onycholysis
This is separation of the distal portion of the nail, causing it to appear white. It arises due to trauma or association with psoriasis and thyrotoxicosis.

Beau's lines
These are transverse white lines due to psychiatric or systemic disease, which cause a temporary cessation of growth. They also occur when chemotherapy is used.

Pitting
Arises due to localised increase in nail growth, classically seen in psoriasis. Pitting may also occur in eczema.

Answer 10

(a) Albinism
Tuberculoid leprosy
Pityriasis versicolor (dark skinned patients)   *(3 marks)*

(b) Type 1 diabetes mellitus
Addison's disease
Pernicious anaemia
Thyroid disease – thyrotoxicosis and myxoedema
                                            (3 marks)

(c) FBC including:
  MCV, U&Es
  Vitamin B12 and folate
  Glucose
Autoantibody screen:
  IF, thyroid   *(4 marks)*

Comment

Vitiligo is a common cause of depigmentation, its incidence varying from 1% in the UK to almost 9% in the Indian sub-continent. It is an autoimmune disorder, but the triggering factors have not as yet been identified. A family history is positive in 33% of cases. Common associations include pernicious anaemia, Addison's disease, thyrotoxicosis, myxoedema and diabetes. On presentation, evidence of other autoimmune disease should always be sought. The lesions of vitiligo are usually symmetrical, and in 50% of cases are apparent before the age of 20 years. They may occur in sites of trauma, such as the knuckles or around a naevus, known as a halo naevus. They may also exhibit the Koebner phenomenon. Other causes of depigmentation include:

- Albinism (partial or complete)
- Phenylketonuria
- Tuberculoid leprosy (associated with anaesthesia)
- Pityriasis versicolor caused by *Malassezia furfur*
- Syphilis
- Ash leaf spots of tuberose sclerosis
- Post-inflammatory depigmentation = *Pityriasis alba* (this occurs in psoriasis and eczema)

ANSWERS

Gastroenterology

Answer 1

(a) (i) Virchow's node and Troisier's sign
   (ii) Nausea
      Vomiting
      Dysphagia
      Haematemesis
      Melaena   *(3 marks)*

(b) (i) Gastroscopy – diagnosis
      Barium meal – diagnosis
   (ii) Endoscopic ultrasound – staging
      CT thorax and abdomen – staging
      Combined FDG–PET/CT scan – staging *(4 marks)*

(c) Iron deficiency
   Vitamin B12 deficiency
   Dumping syndrome
   Alkaline reflux oesophagitis
   Anastomotic stricture
   Vitamin D deficiency/osteomalacia   *(3 marks)*

Comment

Gastric carcinoma is common in the UK, its incidence being approximately one-quarter that of colorectal cancer. Most patients are asymptomatic until local invasion or distant metastasis has occurred. In Japan, where the disease affects up to 10% of the population, a screening programme has resulted in a substantial proportion of diagnoses occurring at an early stage. In the UK, where the lower incidence makes screening impractical, most patients present with inoperable disease. The typical features are as described above. Back pain is a sinister sign, implying local direct invasion. In addition, gastric carcinoma is particularly associated with acanthosis nigricans and dermatomyositis, which occur as paraneoplastic manifestations.

Gastroscopy is the investigation of choice for confirming the diagnosis. Anti-secretory medications should ideally be stopped for a fortnight before the procedure. Barium imaging is also effective at detecting gastric tumours, particularly linitis plastica, but gastroscopy is preferred because it allows simultaneous biopsy. Once the diagnosis has been confirmed, a CT scan of the thorax and abdomen is used in staging for the purposes of planning treatment. FDG-PET (18F-fluorodeoxyglucose positron emission tomography) scanning offers little benefit over CT in terms of prediction of recurrence, but combined PET/CT scanners are more sensitive than CT alone at detecting distant metastasis and so are likely to be used more as their availability increases. If no evidence of metastasis is found, endoscopic ultrasound is used to determine the extent of local spread and, hence, whether the primary tumour is resectable.

Surgical resection with extensive lymphadenectomy offers the only hope of a cure. Total gastrectomy is performed for proximal tumours whereas a partial gastrectomy is possible for distal lesions. Whilst the role of adjuvant and neoadjuvant chemotherapy remains the subject of investigation, palliative chemotherapy is available for inoperable tumours.

Answer 2

(a) Clinical features:
>   No impact pain on swallowing, weight loss or cachexia
>   No cervical adenopathy or anaemia
>
> Investigations:
>   Barium swallow and/or
>   Oesophagoscopy and mucosal biopsy   *(3 marks)*

(b) (i) By oesophageal manometry: a pressure transducer
on a lead is swallowed and records the intra-
luminal and sphincter pressures during swallowing
By video fluoroscopy of swallow   *(2 marks)*

(ii) Achalasia of the cardia (cardiospasm)
Degenerative changes in vagal innervation and
muscular hypertrophy of the lower third of the
oesophagus producing a functional obstruction
(2 marks)

(c) Forceful dilatation of the lower oesophageal sphincter
with a hydrostatic balloon under imaging. Endoscopic
injection of botulinum toxin is an alternative. Failure of
conservative measures is an indication for
Cardiomyotomy (Heller's operation), often performed
laparoscopically.   *(3 marks)*

Comment

In patients with dysphagia, a malignant lesion must be excluded as
a first step. Inflammatory strictures due to acid reflux from hiatus
hernia and accidental ingestion of corrosives in children are more
frequently encountered. Myasthenia gravis or motor neurone
disease may present with dysphagia due to a defect in
neuromuscular transmission. Other causes are progressive
systemic sclerosis, some connective tissue disorders and Chagas'
disease (American trypanosomiasis). Oesophageal candidiasis,
which is readily diagnosed on endoscopy, is frequently regarded as
an AIDS-defining illness and an indication for immunological
screening.

Answer 3

(a) Hiatus hernia with reflux oesophagitis
The lower oesophageal sphincter and the sphincter
mechanism of the crura of the diaphragm are
incompetent, resulting in equalisation of intra-gastric
and oesophageal pressures, producing reflux of gastric
contents into the oesophagus   *(3 marks)*

(b) Oesophageal pH monitoring: a pH probe is placed in the distal oesophagus and acid exposure is monitored in the ambulatory state and at rest. The patient's symptoms are correlated with the actual recording of acid reflux episodes

Acid perfusion (Bernstein) test: symptoms of acid reflux may be reproduced by dripping dilute acid via a nasogastric tube into the distal oesophagus   *(3 marks)*

(c) General measures:

Liquid or chewable antacids (aluminium or magnesium hydroxide 30 ml, 30 min after meals and at bedtime).

Alginic acid antacids (Gaviscon® 10 ml, 30 min after meals and at bedtime).

Elevate head of bed on blocks.

Avoid alcohol, smoking, fatty and spicy food, and food or drink before bed time.

Lose weight

Proton pump inhibitors (PPIs) now form the basis of treatment in the majority of patients with gastro-oesophageal reflux disease (GORD). Severe cases may also require promotility agents and intractable cases, surgical fundoplication may be warranted. All cases should have *H. Pylori* excluded and treated where identified with triple therapy (two antibiotic agents and a PPI).   *(4 marks)*

Comment

Gastro-oesophageal reflux disease is usually associated with a sliding hernia, which interferes with normal oesophageal clearance by acting as a fluid trap. Endoscopic changes in the lower oesophagus range from shallow linear erosions to confluent ulcers to complete mucosal destruction (grades I to IV). Metaplastic changes to columnar epithelium of the lower oesophagus (Barrett's oesophagus) are produced by severe chronic reflux and are associated with the development of an adenocarcinoma.

Answer 4

(a) Peptic ulcer disease   *(2 marks)*

(b) OGD or barium meal examination
Visualisation or imaging of the ulcer in the stomach or
duodenum, with associated deformity or scarring of
the pyloroduodenum. The amount of gastric residue
and the volume of the stomach may suggest delayed
gastric emptying due to pyloric stenosis caused by the
ulcer   *(3 marks)*

(c) In symptomatic disease, where there is no evidence of
H. pylori infection, PPIs such as omeprazole (now
available over the counter), esomeprazole, lansoprazole
or pantoprazole may be given. Other drugs used in this
group of patient include H_2 antagonists, bismuth
colloid, sucralfate (particularly used for biliary reflux)
and symptomatic antacid agents such as aluminium
and magnesium solutions.

For those with identified *H. pylori* infection, a one week
course of 'triple therapy' should be given. This includes
two antibiotic agents e.g. amoxicillin, clarithromycin,
metronidazole and tinidazole with a PPI or H2
antagonist.   *(5 marks)*

Comment

The diagnosis and management of upper GI inflammation and
peptic ulcer disease was revolutionised by the introduction of reliable
endoscopy and the discovery of *H. pylori* in the 1980s. *H. pylori* has
now been implicated in the development of upper GI inflammation,
peptic ulcer disease (60% of gastric ulcers, 90% of duodenal ulcers)
and upper GI malignancies including gastric carcinoma.

Management of these conditions should now include

(a) Advice around lifestyle measures – avoiding alcohol excess, NSAIDs and spicy foods.
(b) Confirmation/exclusion of the presence of *H. pylori*
(c) Symptomatic relief and eradication therapy of *H. pylori* (when present).
(d) Maintenance therapy (where indicated) with low dose PPI or H_2 antagonist.

Answer 5

(a) (i) Malabsorption and steatorrhoea are found in:
　　　　Blind loop syndrome with bacterial overgrowth
　　　　Coeliac disease
　　　　Pancreatic enzyme deficiency
　　　　Bile salt deficiency
　　　　Tropical sprue　　　　　　　　　　　*(3 marks)*
　　(ii) Duodenal biopsy showing
　　　　Mucosal flattening; total/partial villous atrophy
　　　　or raised anti-endomysial antibody titres
　　　　　　　　　　　　　　　　　　　　　(2 marks)

(b) (i) Coeliac disease (gluten-induced enteropathy)
　　　　　　　　　　　　　　　　　　　　　(2 marks)
　　(ii) Small bowel lymphoma/carcinoma
　　　　Dermatitis herpetiformis　　　　　*(3 marks)*

Comment

Steatorrhoea implies malabsorption of fat, with faecal fat excretion in excess of 6 g/day, and signifies an inability to absorb a significant amount of the dietary constituents. The diagnosis in this patient involves distinguishing between an enteropathy and other causes of steatorrhoea. In coeliac disease there is mucosal sensitivity to wheatgerm, barley, rye and, occasionally, oats. The resulting malabsorption involves not only fat and fat-soluble vitamins, but also minerals and water-soluble vitamins. Other causes of malabsorption are obstructive jaundice, pancreatitis, inflammatory bowel disease and overgrowth of bowel organisms.

Treatment is aimed at the cause. In obstructive jaundice bile flow is surgically re-established; pancreatic exocrine insufficiency is treated with pancreatic extract. Acute exacerbations of Crohn's disease and ulcerative colitis are treated with aminosalicylates or sulphasalazine with the addition of immunosuppression (azathioprine) and steroids (prednisolone). Bacterial overgrowth in bowel is encountered in severe malnutrition and is treated with antibiotics and an initial elemental diet.

Answer 6

(a) Ulcerative colitis
Crohn's disease
Infective colitis (campylobacter/amoebic colitis, bacillary dysentery, pseudomembranous colitis)
Ischaemic colitis
Diverticulitis   (3 marks)

(b) (i) Acute ulcerative colitis   (1 mark)
(ii) Perforation
Haemorrhage
Toxic megacolon   (3 marks)

(c) Bedrest with close monitoring of clinical parameters
Nasogastric aspiration
IV rehydration
IV steroids (±azathioprine)
IV antibiotics
Blood transfusion (if anaemic)
Surgery for progressive toxicity, severe haemorrhage
or toxic megacolon   (3 marks)

Comment
The diagnosis of inflammatory bowel disease is usually obvious from a history of relapses and remissions, with progressive deterioration in symptoms, culminating in an acute episode. In ulcerative colitis the rectal mucosa is usually involved, with a variable proximal colonic extension, whilst Crohn's disease mainly involves the distal small bowel, with occasional colonic involvement. However, in 10% of

cases of colitis a definitive diagnosis of either ulcerative colitis or Crohn's disease is not possible. Inflammatory bowel disease is treated by oral aminosalicylates or sulphasalazine. During acute exacerbations intravenous steroids (hydrocortisone) are administered with antibiotics when the risks of complications are high in severe disease. More recently the monoclonal antibody therapy Infiximab, (an anti-tumour necrosis factor antibody (anti-TNF α)) has been successful in severe relapsing disease. However, for the vast majority of sufferers dietary measures alone or with a maintenance dose of aminosalicylates is sufficient to keep the disease in remission.

Long-term colonoscopic surveillance is required for ulcerative colitis in remission due to predisposition to adenocarcinoma.

Answer 7

(a) (i) Diarrhoea, abdominal pain, weight loss, fever, malaise, lethargy, anorexia, nausea, vomiting
(2 marks)

   (ii) Biliary – pericholangitis (19%), calculi
   Kidney – oxalate stone (30%)
   Joints – sacroiliitis (15%–18%), monoarticular arthritis (14%)
   Eye – uveitis (4%)
   Skin – erythema nodosum; pyoderma gangrenosum
   (2 marks)

(b) IV rehydration and electrolyte correction
IV or oral corticosteroid therapy to control the inflammatory exacerbation
Oral aminosalicylates or sulphasalazine for induction and maintenance of remission
Oral immunosuppression (azathioprine) to maintain steroid-induced remission
Oral or IV antibiotic therapy (metronidazole with a cephalosporin or cotrimoxazole) to counter bacterial infection
Bowel rest with total parenteral nutrition or elemental diet
Correct anaemia if present
(3 marks)

(c) Surgery is reserved for complications of the disease: bowel stenosis, fistulation or perforation, abscess formation and rarely haemorrhage. Eighty per cent of patients may require bowel resection at some stage of their disease *(3 marks)*

Comment

Crohn's disease is a chronic mucosal inflammation of uncertain aetiology affecting any part of the gastrointestinal tract. Characteristic microvascular abnormalities have been demonstrated in the lamina propria. Focal arteritis and arterial occlusion lead to haemorrhage and tissue ischaemia with new vessel formation which is thought to be initiated by cytokines and angiogenesis tissue factors. The disease may be confined to one segment of bowel, manifest as multiple skip lesions, or involve the entire small and/or large bowel. The affected bowel is thickened and narrowed, with ulceration and fissuring of the mucosa. There may be associated fistulae and abscess formation. These, along with significant bowel stenosis, require surgical measures to eradicate infection or to restore bowel continuity. The long-term risk of bowel cancer is negligible in Crohn's disease, unlike ulcerative colitis.

Answer 8

(a) (i) B-cell lymphoma of the bowel
Lymphoid hyperplasia of the bowel
Kaposi's sarcoma of the bowel *(2 marks)*

(ii) Cytomegalovirus
Microsporidium or *Cryptosporidium parvum*
Mycobacterium avium intercellulare *(3 marks)*

(b) (i) Plain abdominal X-ray
CT scan of abdomen
Barium enema (for large bowel obstruction)

(2 marks)

(ii) 'Drip and suck' regime to reduce bowel activity
and allow the lymphoidal enlargement causing the
obstruction to regress
The presence of an intussusception causing acute
obstruction requires early surgical relief

(3 marks)

Comment

Due to their suppressed immunity, patients with AIDS are prone to
recurrent bowel infections from a wide variety of pathogens.
Treatment of the atypical bowel infections with antibiotics is
prolonged, and these patients are susceptible to relapses and
recurrent infections. Acute or chronic intussusception may be
produced by lymphatic hyperplasia or a lymphoma. The diagnosis is
often delayed due to the non-specific nature of the symptoms and to
the extensive differential diagnoses of abdominal pathology in these
patients. The early use of CT in diagnosing bowel obstruction
should forestall complications of bowel ischaemia and peritonitis.

Answer 9

(a) (i) Contact bleeding with mucosal friability
Mucosal ulceration
Mucosal granuloma (amoeboma)   *(3 marks)*

(ii) Serology: amoebic fluorescent antibody titres and
precipitating antibody titres may be elevated
Microscopy: examination of wet smears of colonic
scrapings for cysts and trophozoites

(2 marks)

(b) Abnormal liver function tests, viz raised serum alkaline
phosphatase
Liver imaging by ultrasound or radionuclide scan

(2 marks)

(c)   Metronidazole or tinidazole
Dihydroemetine or chloroquine
Diloxanide furoate (furamide)   *(3 marks)*

Comment

Amoebiasis is common in the tropics and is an important cause of imported fever in Britain. It is transmitted in the encysted form via the oro-faecal route and produces a chronic infection of the large bowel. Pain in the right iliac fossa may simulate acute appendicitis, or chronic diarrhoea, and passage of blood-stained mucus may simulate ulcerative colitis. Granuloma formation may be palpable in the rectum or produce a filling defect in the colon on barium enema and must be distinguished from a carcinoma. Hepatic amoebiasis may present without a history of bowel symptoms. A swinging pyrexia and an enlarged, tender liver with shoulder-tip pain are characteristic of abscess formation. The latter responds well to chemotherapy but may require repeated ultrasound-guided aspiration to aid resolution.

Answer 10

(a)   (i)   Chronic pancreatitis   *(1 mark)*
       (ii) Moderate elevation of serum amylase
            titres   *(1 mark)*

(b)   Destruction of the exocrine pancreatic tissue leads to a fall in digestive enzyme secretion resulting in malabsorption. Progressive destruction of the islets of Langerhans of the pancreas leads to diabetes mellitus   *(3 marks)*

(c)   Exocrine enzyme insufficiency is treated by oral
      pancreatic enzyme supplements, the dose of which is
      titrated to reduce steatorrhoea and bowel frequency.
      A neutral duodenal pH to optimise the effect of the
      supplements is achieved by antacids or H2 receptor
      blockers in those that respond poorly
      Endocrine (insulin) insufficiency is treated by soluble
      insulin, as oral hypoglycaemic agents are usually
      ineffective
      General measures include alcohol rehabilitation,
      supervision of analgesic use and diet   *(5 marks)*

Comment

A nutritious and balanced diet, with fat-soluble vitamins (suitably
adjusted for diabetics), with abstinence from alcohol, are the
mainstay of treatment. Pancreatic pain is difficult to treat; whilst
abstinence is essential to reduce the frequency and severity of
attacks, analgesics, frequently narcotic agents, may have to be
resorted to for pain relief. Percutaneous nerve block (coeliac plexus
block) with phenol may be tried if the above measures fail. Over a
ten-year period, about one-third of patients obtain relief of pain
without surgical treatment, and the pain is reduced in a further
one-third. The remainder have progressive symptoms, with a 50%
survival over this period. Surgery in this group takes the form of
internal pancreatic duct drainage or pancreatic resection, but is of
little value in the patient who cannot abstain from alcohol.

Answer 11

(a)   Yellow discoloration of abdominal skin
      Ascites
      Splenomegaly
      Spider naevi
      Caput medusae
      Skin bruising
      Purpuric rash   *(3 marks)*

(b) Raised plasma bilirubin: unconjugated fraction signifies extent of liver damage
Low total plasma proteins and albumin: diminished liver synthesis
Raised alanine and aspartate amino-transferases: both raised in liver disease; alanine transferase more specific in liver damage
Raised gamma-glutamyl transferase: specific for liver damage; distinguishes from bone disease
Raised plasma globulin fraction: indicates underlying liver inflammation, eg hepatitis B infection
Raised alkaline phosphatase: non-specific for liver disease
Raised urinary bilirubin: indicates cholestasis due to hepatic inflammation   *(4 marks)*

(c) Gastrointestinal haemorrhage as a result of chronic liver disease (cirrhosis) is due to:
Portal hypertension leading to gastro-oesophageal varices
Increased incidence of peptic ulceration
Coagulopathy   *(3 marks)*

Comment

The main objectives of treating patients with cirrhosis are to ensure good nutritional status, manage chronic cholestasis and treat complications such as ascites, portal hypertension, hepatic encephalopathy, renal failure and infection. The prognosis in cirrhosis is dependent on the extent of liver damage as reflected by liver function. There is a 50% five-year survival when the patient presents early with satisfactory liver compensation. The prognosis is favourable where the cause is correctable, as in alcoholism, haemochromatosis and Wilson's disease.

Answer 12

(a) The clinical spectrum ranges from non-specific
     symptoms without detectable abnormality to acute
     liver failure or advanced cirrhosis
     Alcoholic hepatitis may be a severe illness, with a tender
     hepatomegaly and cholestatic jaundice
     It may resolve completely if the insult is removed and
     no lasting liver damage is present
     Irreversible liver damage leads to cirrhosis, which may
     present as portal hypertension, ascites or encephalopathy,
     characterising end-stage liver disease   *(4 marks)*

(b) Early liver lesion: fatty change/infiltration (reversible)
     Alcoholic hepatitis: inflammatory cell infiltration with
     foci of hepatocyte necrosis
     Mallory's hyaline: pink-staining inclusion bodies found
     in inflamed hepatocytes
     Central hyaline sclerosis: fibrosis around central veins
     Cirrhosis: initially micro-nodular progressing to
     macro-nodular cirrhosis
     Mild siderosis: iron deposits in hepatocytes   *(3 marks)*

(c) Abstinence from alcohol is an important prognostic
     factor as it promotes complete resolution of fatty
     change, halts the progressive necrosis of hepatocytes,
     and improves health and survival
     Progressive alcoholic hepatitis results in a significant
     mortality from acute liver failure; those who recover may
     progress to cirrhosis, in which hepatocyte destruction
     and fibrosis of the liver produce end-stage liver disease
     Variceal bleeding, ascites, encephalopathy and hepato-
     cellular carcinoma are grave complications of alcoholic
     cirrhosis   *(3 marks)*

Comment

Alcoholic liver disease is common in many societies, and the extent
and severity of the liver damage caused is directly related to the
duration of alcohol abuse and the amount consumed daily. It is

frequently difficult to obtain a history of excessive drinking from the patient and it is useful to question the relatives. Peripheral macrocytosis and a raised gamma-glutamyl transferase suggest the diagnosis. Definitive treatment of irreversible alcoholic liver damage is by liver transplantation, and in order to make this treatment cost-effective, complete abstinence must be demonstrated by the patient.

Answer 13

(a) Parenteral via peripheral or central venous access
Enteral, ie via the gut   *(2 marks)*

(b) BMI = weight in kilogrammes/(height in metres)^2
FBC, U&Es, glucose, albumin, calcium, magnesium
Trace elements, eg zinc
Ferritin, vitamin B12 and folate   *(4 marks)*

(c) Is the gut working? Severe gut dysmotility is a
contraindication to the use of enteral feeding,
eg paralytic ileus
Catabolic states, eg sepsis, burns – require increased
nitrogen load
Renal impairment – limit protein (nitrogen) content
and volume of the feed
Liver failure – limit protein content
Diabetes mellitus – limit carbohydrate content and
requires insulin cover
Duration of morbidity – if prolonged requires
long-term enteral feeding   *(4 marks)*

Comment

On admission to hospital all patients should have a simple nutritional assessment. The patient's present weight and height should be recorded and their 'usual' weight (and when last weighed) should also be ascertained. Any patient who has, by these simple criteria, lost 10% of their 'usual' weight is in need of nutritional support. In deciding what form of nutritional help they require, one simple rule must be followed: 'If the gut is working, use it'. If the patient is relatively well and is able to eat and drink, build-up drinks should be used. These contain approximately 500 kilocalories, essential vitamins and trace elements. They are most often used to supplement an inadequate diet. In more severe cases, such as dysphagia secondary to stroke, bulbar palsy or motor neurone disease, gastrostomy or jejunostomy feeding is used. This is also the first-line choice of patients who require long-term feeding. When the bowel is dysfunctional, eg mechanical obstruction, high output diarrhoea or in short bowel syndrome, parenteral feeding is indicated. Peripheral venous feeding is used to supplement the diet for short periods of time. It is limited due to the phlebitic nature of certain elements of the feeds. In prolonged and debilitating illness, feeding is through tunnelled central venous lines and the nutritional contents tailored to the individual needs.

Answer 14

(a) Oesophageal varices   *(1 mark)*
Oesophagitis, Mallory–Weiss tear, gastritis, peptic ulcer disease   *(2 marks)*

(b) FBC, U&Es, glucose, LFTs, clotting screen, crossmatch (at least six units)   *(3 marks)*

(c) Lie patient head down (in left lateral position if vomiting)
Endotracheal intubation if unable to protect airway
IV access – one large bore cannula in each forearm
If any signs of shock insert central venous line
Start colloid infusion or, if severe bleed, start blood transfusion with Rhesus O negative blood
Start blood transfusion with crossmatched blood, FFP and platelets transfusion as required
IV Terlipressin 2 mg bolus then 1 mg every 4 hours
Give IV vitamin K if deranged INR
Arrange upper GI endoscopy and urgent surgical assessment
If ongoing variceal bleeding consider insertion of Sengstaken–Blakemore tube   *(4 marks)*

Comment

The prognosis in acute upper GI bleeds has not changed since the 1960s despite the advent of endoscopy and earlier surgical intervention. Overall mortality is 8%–12% but in specialist units it can be as low as 4%. Mortality rate increases with age, to over 50% in the over 75-year-olds. (The ageing population is thought to be one of the reasons for the lack of prognostic improvement.) The principal prognostic indicator in this group is re-bleeding. In patients with concurrent peptic ulcer disease, the endoscopic appearances of fresh blood clot or visible vessels in the ulcer crater both signify a high risk. Identifying these patients and treating them aggressively improves their prognosis.

Oesophageal varices arise due to portal hypertension from chronic liver disease. Variceal bleeds tend to be torrential and are exacerbated by coagulopathy secondary to loss of vitamin-K-dependent factors and thrombocytopenia. These carry a poor prognosis, with 50% of patients dying within six weeks of their first bleed. Emergency treatment includes protection of the airway, fluid resuscitation, endoscopy and injection or banding of the varices. Terlipressin, a vasopressin analogue, is used to constrict the splanchnic circulation and hence reduce portal venous pressure. Terlipressin (Glypressin®) has replaced vasopressin, which also constricts the coronary vasoconstriction, causing cardiac ischaemia. The somatostatin analogue, octreotide, is also used. The somatostatin analogue, octreotide, is also used.

Transjugular intrahepatic portal systemic shunt (TIPSS) may be used for torrential variceal bleeds. This is a stented shunt between the portal and hepatic veins, which leads to decompression of the portal system.

Answer 15

(a) Dyspeptic history or ingestion of alcohol, steroids and non-steroidal anti-inflammatory agents are linked to peptic ulcer disease
A violent bout of vomiting or retching is linked to an oesophageal mucosal tear
Anorexia, weight loss, malaise may be associated with gastric cancer
History of liver disease is linked to variceal haemorrhage   *(4 marks)*

(b) OGD   *(2 marks)*

(c) Endoscopic biopsies for histological confirmation
FBC: for anaemia
LFTs: to assess liver function
U&Es: to assess renal function
Liver imaging for metastatic tumour deposits
Definitive treatment: a form of gastrectomy or a by-pass if unresectable with/without radiotherapy/chemotherapy   *(4 marks)*

Comment

Fluid resuscitation is the first priority in managing acute upper gastrointestinal haemorrhage. Two large-bore intravenous cannulae should be inserted, blood samples obtained and one to two litres crystalloid solution administered. The targets for pulse and systolic blood pressure are <100 beats per minute and >100 mmHg respectively. Urine output should be maintained at >30 ml/hr. Vital signs should be recorded frequently (at least every fifteen minutes in severe cases). Blood transfusion may be necessary if the haemoglobin is <10 g/dl. Intravenous infusion of omeprazole reduces the risk of rebleeding and the duration of hospital admission. If variceal bleeding is a possibility, terlipressin should also be administered. The patient is kept nil by mouth pending endoscopy, which may provide a diagnosis and also allow direct haemostasis.

Nephrology

Answer 1

(a) Fibromuscular dysplasia *(1 mark)*

(b) Low K^+ and high HCO_3^- because a low glomerular filtration rate results in renin release from granular cells of the juxtaglomerular apparatus. Renin catalyses the conversion of angiotensinogen to angiotensin I, which in turn is converted (by angiotensin converting enzyme) to angiotensin II, a potent vasoconstrictor and the main stimulus to aldosterone release. Aldosterone acts at the distal convoluted tubule to promote Na^+ retention at the expense of K^+ and H^+ ions. *(5 marks)*

(c) Stop the ACE inhibitor
Recheck the U&E
Full history, including family history of hypertension, and examination, including for renal and other bruits
Magnetic resonance angiography of the renal arteries
Balloon angioplasty stenoses if possible *(4 marks)*

Comment

A secondary cause should be sought when hypertension occurs in the young or when it is severe, and/or resistant to treatment. Renal artery stenosis should particularly be suspected in patients presenting with flash pulmonary oedema or renal failure precipitated by ACE inhibitor treatment. Renal ultrasound is used first to exclude other structural abnormalities associated with hypertension, such as polycystic kidney disease. Magnetic resonance angiography is the method of choice for imaging the renal arteries directly, since it is sensitive and non-invasive. Other options include arterial Doppler ultrasound, which is operator-dependent, and intra-arterial digital subtraction angiography, which is considered the gold standard investigation but which involves considerable risk for the patient.

The commonest cause of renal artery stenosis is atherosclerosis. Unfortunately, culprit lesions are seldom solitary, so it is uncommon for angioplasty, with or without stent, to effect a cure of hypertension, although it sometimes improves renal function. In contrast, fibromuscular dysplasia, which usually presents in young women, may often be cured by angioplasty, allowing complete cessation of antihypertensive treatment.

ACE inhibitors (and angiotensin II receptor antagonists) may cause acute renal failure in patients with renal artery stenosis. This occurs because, in the presence of critical stenoses, glomerular filtration pressure is maintained by intense constriction of efferent arterioles under the influence of angiotensin II. If the constriction is prevented by ACE inhibition or angiotensin II receptor blockade, afferent flow is insufficient to maintain intraglomerular pressure, with catastrophic results.

Answer 2

(a) Ascending urinary sepsis affecting the grafted kidney
Gentamicin nephrotoxicity
Tacrolimus nephrotoxicity
Renal graft rejection   *(2 marks)*

(b) Prednisolone: binds to the glucocorticoid receptor to alter gene transcription in inflammatory pathways
Tacrolimus: calcineurin inhibitor
Mycophenolate mofetil: blocks lymphocyte purine synthesis   *(4 marks)*

(c) Basiliximab (anti-CD25 antibody): hypersensitivity reactions, cytokine release syndrome
Daclizumab (anti-Tac antibody): hypersensitivity reactions
Sirolimus: hyperlipidaemia, thrombocytopenia, neutropenia   *(4 marks)*

Comment

The purpose of immunosuppressive therapy in renal transplantation is to prevent T-cell-mediated graft rejection. Patients are thus vulnerable to a range of opportunistic infections and tumours, similar to that seen in advanced HIV disease. The risk is greatest during the first six months after transplantation, when immunosuppression is maximal. In addition to this, each individual drug has its own range of adverse effects:

Drug	Typical side-effects
Glucocorticoids (corticosteroids)	
Prednisolone	hypertension
Methylprednisolone	glucose intolerance/diabetes
	weight gain
	dyslipidaemia
	osteoporosis
	suppression of inflammatory signs and symptoms of sepsis, eg from bowel perforation
Calcineurin-blocking drugs	
Ciclosporin	nephrotoxicity
Tacrolimus	glucose intolerance
	neurotoxicity
	hypertrichosis (ciclosporin)
	gingival hypertrophy (ciclosporin)
Purine synthesis inhibitors	
Azathioprine	abdominal colic, diarrhoea
Mycophenolate	myelosuppression
mTOR inhibitors	
Sirolimus	hypercholesterolaemia
	hypertriglyceridaemia
	thrombotic thrombocytopenic purpura
Anti-lymphocyte antibodies	
Basiliximab	hypersensitivity (rare)
Daclizumab	

Answer 3

(a) Erythropoietin deficiency secondary to renal failure
Haematinic deficiencies secondary to repeated
phlebotomy and small volume blood loss at the end of
dialysis sessions   *(3 marks)*

(b) Recombinant erythropoietin
Iron replacement (usually parenteral)
Vitamin B12 replacement
Folate replacement   *(4 marks)*

(c) Amyloidosis
Secondary or tertiary hyperparathyroidism
Dyslipidaemia
Hyperhomocystinaemia   *(3 marks)*

Comment

Renal replacement therapy for chronic renal failure may be achieved
with haemodialysis, peritoneal dialysis or renal transplant. Each
technique has advantages and disadvantages, but hypertension,
cardiovascular disease, anaemia and amyloidosis are particularly
common in haemodialysis-treated patients. Hypertension is
frequently a factor in the development of renal failure. It may also be
exacerbated by anaemia and haemodialysis, in particular by chronic
volume overload and frequent large swings in circulating blood
volume. Hypertension itself is a risk factor for the development of
cardiovascular disease, which is the major cause of death of patients
with chronic renal failure. Haemodialysis also causes
hyperhomocystinuria, dyslipidaemia and low-grade inflammation,
all of which contribute to the risk of cardiovascular disease.

Dialysis-related amyloidosis results from the accumulation of
$\beta2$-microglobulin. This is a small protein (part of the class 1 major
histocompatibility complex) that is freely filtered across normal
glomeruli but poorly cleared by haemodialysis. Polymerisation of the
protein results in amyloid deposition, typically causing carpal tunnel
syndrome. A destructive arthropathy with bone cysts may also occur.

Answer 4

(a) Acute left-sided pyelonephritis   *(1 mark)*

(b) FBC, U&Es, glucose
Blood cultures
MSU; urinalysis
Plain AXR   *(4 marks)*

(c) Immediate management:
    IV access
    IV fluids, antiemetics and analgesia
    IV broad-spectrum antibiotics – gentamicin and
    cefuroxime
Secondary investigation:
    USS of kidneys, ureter and bladder
    IVU
    Consider micturating cystogram to exclude
    vesicoureteric reflux   *(5 marks)*

Comment

Pyelonephritis is an infective condition of the kidney, that may present in an acute or chronic manner. In the acute form, the patient presents with loin pain, fever, rigors, and nausea and vomiting. Severe cases with bilateral renal involvement may present with acute renal failure. Treatment should include symptom relief and intravenous antibiotics, particularly gentamicin.

Chronic pyelonephritis, has recently been re-termed 'reflux nephropathy', as it is principally caused by chronic vesicoureteric reflux. This condition arises due to abnormalities of the ureters, which in turn lead to retrograde urinary regurgitation through the vesicoureteric junction. The kidneys therefore become scarred, atrophic and, on imaging, are small and have classically blunted calyces. The diagnosis may be made coincidentally on routine abdominal ultrasound scan, as it is often asymptomatic for many years. Classically it presents in childhood with recurrent urinary tract infections and loin pain. Other presenting features are renal failure, persistent proteinuria, hypertension and renal calculi.

Treatment of vesicoureteric reflux largely depends on the stage of the disease at presentation. In children that present early with moderate to severe disease, there is a place for corrective surgery. In later presentations, or in mild to moderate disease, there is little evidence to suggest that surgery changes overall outcome, and these patients should be managed conservatively, with careful monitoring of their renal function and low-dose prophylactic antibiotics.

Answer 5

(a) Bilateral hydronephrosis
Bilateral renal tumours, eg renal carcinoma *(2 marks)*

(b) Haematuria – associated with bleeding into cysts, recurrent UTIs and, more rarely, renal carcinoma
Recurrent UTIs
Loin pain – this may be due to infection, bleeding into cysts and to the renal enlargement, which causes a non-specific, dull loin pain
Hypertension
Chronic renal failure
Renal carcinoma – this is a rare complication *(5 marks)*

(c) Treat hypertension and UTIs
Regular follow-up in renal outpatients to monitor renal function
In end-stage disease they require dialysis and renal transplantation
Genetic counselling for patient and family *(3 marks)*

Comment

Polycystic kidney disease is the commonest inherited disorder to affect the kidney, and is responsible for 8%–10% of end-stage renal failure seen in the UK. It has two modes of inheritance, autosomal dominant (classically termed adult polycystic kidney disease) and infantile disease, which is an autosomal recessive disorder. The abnormal gene locus (PKD1), responsible for the majority of the adult cases, is located on chromosome 16 and encodes the polycystin-1 gene; another locus (PKD2) on chromosome 4 encodes the polycystin-2 gene. Infantile disease is due to mutations in the fibrocystin gene on chromosome 6.

Both disorders are associated with cystic disease in several other intra-abdominal organs, including the liver, pancreas, spleen and ovaries (this should not be confused with polycystic ovary syndrome). The infantile form is also associated with hepatic fibrosis and portal hypertension.

Although it is occasionally discovered in childhood, the adult form usually presents in the third to fourth decades, with local and systemic complications. Systemic complications and associations include:

- Hypertension (it is important to control hypertension as this accelerates renal failure)
- Polycythaemia (due to increased erythropoietin secretion)
- Liver cysts (these occur in 70% of patients)
- Berry aneurysms (patients present with subarachnoid haemorrhage; all patients should be asked about a family history of sudden death or stroke)
- Mitral valve prolapse

Answer 6

(a) Hypoalbuminaemia < 30 g/l
Proteinuria > 3–5 g/24 hours
Peripheral oedema   *(3 marks)*

(b) Fusion of the podocytes, with no other associated glomerular changes   *(2 marks)*

(c) U&E, eGFR
Urine protein excretion – 24 hour collection or protein
Creatinine ratio on spot morning sample
Serum albumin
USS of the kidneys, ureters and bladder
Renal biopsy
Therapeutic management – high-dose oral steroids
cyclophosphamide (in severe cases)   *(5 marks)*

CHAPTER 10 – ANSWERS

Comment

Minimal change nephropathy is the commonest cause of an idiopathic nephrotic syndrome, accounting for 70%–80% in children, 60% in adolescents and 25% in adults. It is not a true glomerulonephritis, and the characteristic fusion of the podocytes seen on electron microscopy is a non-specific sign which occurs in many other nephrotic states.

The pathogenesis of the disorder remains unclear, but it is thought to be an immune-mediated disease as it responds so well to immunosuppression with high-dose steroids or cyclophosphamide. It is associated with Hodgkin's lymphoma, and is seen to resolve with successful treatment of the lymphoma. In adolescents (more than ten years old) and adults it is recommended that the diagnosis is confirmed on renal biopsy. This is important as the disease does not progress to chronic renal failure and the patient may then be assured of a good prognosis.

Answer 7

(a) Drugs – prescribed medications, eg gold salts and illicit drug abuse
Infection, eg streptococcus, malaria
Systemic vasculitides – SLE, PAN, Wegener's granulomatosis
Diabetes mellitus
Amyloidosis
Allergic reactions   *(3 marks)*

(b) FBC, U&Es, glucose
ESR
Cholesterol
Autoantibody screen – ANCA, ANF, rheumatoid factor
24-hour urine collection for creatinine clearance and protein estimation
USS of the kidneys
Renal biopsy   *(5 marks)*

(c) Renal failure
Renal vein thrombosis
Sepsis *(2 marks)*

Comment

The glomerulonephritides are a heterogeneous group of disorders
that are characterised according to their pathological features
under light and electron microscopy, and by immunofluorescent
staining. These features are a reflection of the glomerular damage
that occurs due to deposition of immune complexes or to
antiglomerular basement membrane antibodies.

Common causes of the glomerulonephritides are:

- Infection (bacterial – streptococci, leprosy, syphilis, infective
  endocarditis; viral – EBV, HBV, HCV; fungal – candidiasis;
  parasitic – malaria, schistosomiasis)
- Drugs (penicillamine, gold salts, ACE inhibitors)
- Autoimmune (SLE, rheumatoid arthritis, thyroid disease)
- Systemic vasculitides (Wegener's granulomatosis, PAN)
- Malignancy (carcinoma of the lung, breast and colon, Hodgkin's
  disease).

Answer 8

(a) Hyperkalaemia
Renal failure
Normochromic, normocytic anaemia *(2 marks)*

(b) Poorly controlled diabetes mellitus
Hypertension
Recent addition of an ACE inhibitor *(3 marks)*

(c) Hospital admission
IV access
Cardiac monitoring
IV 15–20 units of soluble insulin with 40–50 ml of 50% dextrose solution
Calcium resonium 15 g tds orally
Consider IV calcium gluconate (cardioprotective)
If the serum potassium does not fall, dialysis is required

(5 marks)

Comment

Diabetic nephropathy principally arises due to microvascular disease, exacerbated by recurrent urinary tract infections and hypertension. The characteristic pathological change is nodular glomerulosclerosis, also called the Kimmelstiel–Wilson lesion. Progression of the nephropathy is readily divided into four categories:

- Hyperperfusion of the kidney associated with glomerular hypertrophy
- Microalbuminuria (this is a marker for both hypertension and the resultant damage to the renal parenchyma)
- Macroalbuminuria (> 300 mg/24 hours – this occurs with progressive deterioration of the glomerular filtration and worsening hypertension)
- Frank renal failure (this may be associated with a nephrotic syndrome)

By maintaining tight normoglycaemic control with insulin, and adding an ACE inhibitor for hypertension and microalbuminuria, it has been shown that the progression of the disease may be retarded and, in some cases, even caused to regress.

Answer 9

(a) Amyloidosis
Drugs, eg NSAIDs and gold salts *(2 marks)*

(b) USS of the kidneys
     Renal biopsy
     Rectal biopsy for amyloid
     24-hour urine collection for protein and creatinine
     clearance   *(3 marks)*

(c) Admit to a specialist renal unit
     Remove exacerbating factors, eg drugs
     Consider CAPD or haemofiltration depending on the
     degree of renal impairment
     Nutritional support – low-protein diet
     Symptomatic relief of rheumatoid symptoms
                                                  (5 marks)

Comment

Renal amyloidosis may arise through primary and secondary
causes of amyloid. It is mainly seen in AA amyloidosis but also
occurs in 50% of AL amyloid. AA amyloid commonly arises
secondary to chronic inflammatory and infective disorders, such
as tuberculosis, rheumatoid arthritis, inflammatory bowel disease
and malignancies, eg renal cell carcinoma.

Patients present with proteinuria, often to nephrotic levels, and
postural hypotension. Ultrasound scan will often reveal normal or
enlarged kidneys, even in end-stage disease, due to the amyloid
infiltration.

Diagnosis is made on renal or rectal biopsy, the latter being a more
simple procedure, with a high sensitivity. Histologically amyloid is
characterised by its ability to bind Congo red, which gives it an
apple green appearance under polarised light.

Answer 10

(a) Polyarteritis nodosa
     Henoch–Schönlein purpura
     Wegener's granulomatosis
     SLE   *(3 marks)*

(b)   c-ANCA, p-ANCA, HBs antigen   *(2 marks)*

(c)   Renal biopsy
Renal angiography
Skin biopsy
Management:
     Immunosuppression – azathioprine and
     cyclophosphamide
     Antihypertensive therapy, eg ACE inhibitors,
     calcium-channel blockers
     Treatment of renal impairment – may require
     dialysis   *(5 marks)*

Comment

The systemic vasculitides are a group of diseases characterised by inflammatory and degenerative changes within the blood vessel wall, causing a secondary systemic disorder, which commonly includes the kidney.

They are classified according to the size of the vessel they affect, and the presence or absence of associated granulomata.

Vessel size	Granuloma formation	No granuloma formation
Large	Giant cell arteritis Takayasu's disease	
Medium		Polyarteritis nodosa
Small	Wegener's granulomatosis Churg–Strauss syndrome	Microscopic polyangiitis Henoch–Schönlein purpura

Polyarteritis nodosa, Wegener's granulomatosis, and microscopic polyangiitis classically cause vasculitic renal damage, with an associated glomerulonephritis and hypertension.

Polyarteritis is characterised by aneurysm formation within the renal vasculature, which is demonstrated by renal angiography.

Unlike the other vasculitides in this group, polyarteritis has no specific immune marker, but in certain subgroups of patients there is an association with the HBs antigen. Clinically, the disease normally presents with non-specific systemic features, such as myalgia, arthralgia, anorexia and low-grade fever. However, in some cases its presentation is dramatic with myocardial infarction, CVA or gastrointestinal haemorrhage.

Treatment is similar for all of the systemic vasculitides, using high-dose steroids and immunosuppressants, such as azathioprine and cyclophosphamide.

Answer 11

(a) Normochromic, normocytic anaemia
     Hypoalbuminaemia
     Hypocalcaemia, hyperphosphataemia   (3 marks)

(b) Blood pressure (lying and standing)
     Urinalysis
     Capillary blood glucose measurement   (3 marks)

(c) (i) Anaemia:
            Exclude iron, vitamin B12 and folate deficiency
            Blood transfusion – if symptomatic
            Consider giving erythropoietin (EPO)
     (ii) Renal impairment:
            Maintain good blood pressure control
            Treat any underlying reversible or exacerbating factors
            Will need dialysis, consider renal transplantation
     (iii) Hypocalcaemia:
            Calcium supplements
            Alfacalcidol
     (iv) Hyperphosphataemia:
            Phosphate binders, eg aluminium hydroxide
                                                    (4 marks)

Comment

Chronic renal failure is defined as an irreversible loss of renal function, characteristically associated with a substantial rise in urea and creatinine, a normochromic, normocytic anaemia, hypocalcaemia and hyperphosphataemia. The anaemia may be secondary to the underlying cause of the renal impairment, drug therapy or to the loss of renal erythropoietin production. The anaemic patient may require erythropoietin replacement, although only some patients benefit from this form of treatment, who are thought to be in a genetically determined subgroup.

The disturbances in calcium/phosphate metabolism result in several effects on the skeleton, known as renal osteodystrophy. Osteomalacia arises due to the defective renal hydroxylation of 25-hydroxy-cholecalciferol (25-OH,D3), which in turn leads to a reduced calcium absorption from the gut. Secondary hyperparathyroidism arises due to this chronic hypocalcaemia, which eventually causes tertiary hyperparathyroidism and leads to a rise in the calcium. Without treatment this hypercalcaemia leads to renal calcification, hypercalciuria and further renal damage through stone formation.

Answer 12

(a) Dehydration leading to pre-renal impairment
Thrombocytopenia
Diabetes mellitus
Possible sepsis
Hyperosmolar pre-coma   *(3 marks)*

(b) Blood tests – clotting screen, including D-dimers and FDPs
Blood cultures
ABGs
MSU
ECG
CXR   *(4 marks)*

(c)   Prerenal: cardiogenic, hypovolaemic and septic shock
      Renal: tubulointerstitial nephritis, glomerulonephritis
      Postrenal (obstructive): stones, tumours, foreign
      bodies   *(3 marks)*

Comment

Acute renal failure is characterised by a rapid deterioration in
glomerular filtration rate, which clinically manifests itself as
oliguria or anuria, and biochemically is reflected by worsening
urea and creatinine.

It is usually classified into prerenal, renal and postrenal
(obstructive) causes:

- Prerenal – this results from hypoperfusion of the kidney due to
  renovascular disease or shock. If the cause remains uncorrected it
  causes acute tubular necrosis. Prerenal failure is usually reversible
  providing the kidneys were functioning normally prior to the
  insult, and the causes are quickly diagnosed and treated
- Renal – examples include: acute tubular necrosis,
  glomerulonephritis, autoimmune disease (rheumatoid arthritis,
  SLE, systemic vasculitides), PAN, Wegener's granulomatosis,
  tubulointerstitial nephritis (sickle cell disease, NSAIDs,
  nephrotoxins), myoglobin, Bence Jones proteins
- Obstructive – this occurs due to internal obstruction or external
  compression of the urinary tract. External compression –
  prostatic enlargement, pelvic and rectal tumours,
  retroperitoneal fibrosis and lymphoma; internal obstruction –
  ureteric stones, pelvicalyceal and ureteric tumours, bladder
  stones and tumours, foreign bodies

Answer 13

(a)   Anion gap = [Na + K] – [chloride + bicarbonate]
                 = [134 + 3.1] – [114 + 12]
                 = 137.1 – 126
                 = 11.1 (normal range 8–16 mmol/l)
                                                      (3 marks)

    (b) Type I – sickle cell disease
          Type II – heavy metal toxicity
          Type IV – Addison's disease   *(3 marks)*

    (c) Diabetic ketoacidosis
          Lactic acidosis
          General management – IV access
          IV fluids
          IV sliding scale of insulin
          Treat underlying cause, eg sepsis
          If new diagnosis:
             Address associated risk factors
             Diabetic education   *(4 marks)*

Comment

Renal tubular acidosis is caused by a heterogeneous group of disorders, and is characterised by hyperchloraemia, a normal anion gap and a metabolic (ie low bicarbonate) acidosis. There are three recognised variants, classified according to the abnormal tubule site.

Type I
Distal hypokalaemic hyperchloraemic acidosis – in this disorder the distal tubules are unable to secrete hydrogen (H^+) ions, which causes secondary hyperaldosteronism and results in the hypokalaemia and hyperchloraemia. Causes include:

- Autoimmune disease (SLE, CAH, Sjögren's syndrome)
- Drugs (NSAIDs, amphotericin)
- Nephrocalcinosis (hyperparathyroidism)
- Obstructive nephropathy

Type II
Proximal hypokalaemic hyperchloraemic acidosis – the principal abnormality in this condition is the inability of the proximal tubules to reabsorb bicarbonate. It may be associated with a generalised defect of reabsorption, known as Fanconi's syndrome, where amino acids, glucose and other ions are also lost in the urine.

Fanconi's syndrome may be inherited as a rare autosomal recessive condition, but is more commonly acquired secondary to myeloma, heavy metal toxicity or drugs.

Type IV

Distal hyperkalaemic hyperchloraemic acidosis – this differs from type I in that there is a generalised distal tubular defect, with an associated reduction in the glomerular filtration rate, and the resulting hyperkalaemia may be life threatening.

Causes include mineralocorticoid deficiency in Addison's disease, adrenalectomy, diabetic nephropathy and obstructive nephropathy, and tubular resistance to mineralocorticoid effects, eg spironolactone.

Type III

Type III is a rare condition which has elements of types I and II. It is now therefore not described as a separate entity.

11

Rheumatology and Connective Tissue Diseases

Answer 1

(a) Gottron's sign *(1 mark)*

(b) (i) Muscle biopsy
Serum antibodies: antisynthetase, eg anti-Jo1
anti-Mi2

(ii) Aspiration pneumonia
Interstitial pulmonary fibrosis *(4 marks)*

(c) Cancer
Chest radiograph
Mammography
Gastroscopy
Flexible sigmoidoscopy *(5 marks)*

Comment

Dermatomyositis is an inflammatory disorder that is twice as common in females as males. It occurs in all age groups but, in older patients, is very strongly associated with the onset of malignancy, particularly gastric carcinoma. Features include:

- Proximal myopathy:
  - Serum creatine kinase elevated up to 50 times the upper limit of normal
  - Muscle biopsy shows perivascular, intrafascicular inflammatory infiltrate

- Rashes:
  - Gottron's sign (a rash over the knuckles that is pathognomonic of the disease)
  - Heliotrope rash (purple discoloration and swelling of the eyelids)
  - Erythematous rash affecting the neck, shoulders ('shawl' sign), hands and face
- Myositis-specific antibodies (positive in one-third of patients):
  - Antisynthetase antibodies (also occur in polymyositis)
  - Anti-Mi2 antibodies (specific to dermatomyositis)
- Lung involvement:
  - Interstitial pulmonary fibrosis
  - Recurrent aspiration pneumonia (resulting from oesophageal weakness)
  - Hypercapnic respiratory failure (as a result of weakness of the diaphragm and intercostal muscles)

Corticosteroids are the first-line treatment but azathioprine, methotrexate and/or cyclophosphamide are frequently necessary. In view of the close association with cancer in all age groups except the very young, a diagnosis of dermatomyositis should prompt a search for evidence of malignant disease, with history-taking and examination being supplemented by limited screening investigations if necessary.

Answer 2

(a) Primary Sjögren's syndrome
Tear formation:　Schirmer's test
　　　　　　　　Rose Bengal staining
Salivary function:　Salivary gland scintigraphy
　　　　　　　　Labial gland biopsy　*(4 marks)*

(b) Artificial tears
Eye ointment (nocturnal)
Tarsorrhaphy or occlusion of the canaliculi (to help retain tear film)
Artificial saliva spray
Prompt treatment of secondary infections:
    conjunctivitis: chloramphenicol drops and ointment.
    oral candidiasis: fluconazole
Hydroxychloroquine may be helpful in treating associated arthritis
Corticosteroids and cytotoxic agents only if systemic symptoms prominent   *(3 marks)*

(c) The patient is of child-bearing age; there is a significant risk of congenital heart block in children of women with anti-Ro and anti-La antibodies   *(3 marks)*

Comment

Sjögren's syndrome may occur independently (primary disease) or in association with other rheumatological disorders (secondary Sjögren's syndrome). It is nine times more common in women than men. Uncomplicated disease, consisting only of keratoconjunctivitis sicca (dry eyes) and xerostomia (dry mouth), may be treated very successfully with topical, symptomatic measures. However, the illness may also present with systemic features including fatigue, weight loss, Raynaud's phenomenon and arthritis.

Schirmer's test, used to demonstrate keratoconjunctivitis sicca, is performed by hooking a small strip of filter paper over the lower eyelid. The rate of wetting of the paper by tear film is a guide to severity. An alternative is to look for epithelial degeneration with Rose Bengal staining. Abnormal laboratory tests in Sjögren's syndrome include elevated ESR, pronounced hypergammaglobulinaemia and positive rheumatoid factor and antinuclear antibodies. Anti-Ro and anti-La antibodies occur in a proportion of patients, and infants born to antibody-positive women are at risk of congenital heart block. Labial salivary gland biopsy, the most definitive diagnostic test, typically reveals periductal and periacinar lymphocytic infiltration.

Infection by HIV-1, HTLV-1 or hepatitis C virus may result in a very similar clinical syndrome. Serological testing for these viruses should therefore form part of the diagnostic work-up.

Answer 3

(a) Septic arthritis and septicaemia
Knee differential: acute gout
acute pseudogout   *(3 marks)*

(b) Staphylococcus aureus bacteraemia emanating from
the chronic leg ulcer   *(2 marks)*

(c) Blood cultures
Joint aspiration – fluid sent for Gram stain, white cell count, culture and polarised light microscopy
X-ray knee
Intravenous antibiotics providing staphylococcal cover, eg flucloxacillin or cefuroxime, or vancomycin if methicillin resistance is likely, with gentamicin
Intravenous fluid resuscitation (with care)
Urgent orthopaedic opinion regarding arthroscopic washout   *(5 marks)*

Comment
Acute septic arthritis in a previously healthy joint usually occurs as a result of haematogenous spread of invasive bacteria, eg from skin ulceration, dental abscess or instrumentation of the bladder or bowel. Presentation is thus frequently complicated by evidence of sepsis syndrome. Blood culture and examination of a synovial fluid aspirate are essential investigations. Synovial fluid appears turbid, as is the case in acute gout or pseudogout, but an absence of uric acid or pyrophosphate crystals on polarised light microscopy excludes these diagnoses.

With appropriate antibiotics and frequent therapeutic joint aspiration, a good outcome may sometimes be obtained. However, arthroscopic washout is often necessary, particularly for hip and shoulder joints, where the risk of avascular necrosis of the femoral and humeral heads, respectively, is very high if treatment is delayed.

When sepsis affects a prosthetic joint, the patient may present with a periarticular abscess or discharging sinus, with pain from a loosened prosthesis, or with an acute arthritis similar to that seen in native joints. Removal of the infected prosthesis is usually necessary, with any planned revision surgery being performed after prolonged antibiotic treatment.

Answer 4

(a) Antiphospholipid syndrome   *(1 mark)*

(b) Lupus anticoagulant ± anticardiolipin antibody
                                                                  (1 mark)

(c) Recurrent or atypical venous thrombosis
     Arterial thrombosis
     Recurrent miscarriage/late fetal loss
     Pre-eclampsia/fetal growth restriction
     Thrombocytopenia   *(3 marks)*

(d) Acutely:
        Anticoagulate with heparin then warfarin
     After recovery:
        Consider life-long anticoagulation
        Assess for features of systemic lupus erythematosus
     Next pregnancy:
        Low-dose aspirin and low-molecular-weight heparin
        from first positive pregnancy test until delivery
                                                                  (5 marks)

Comment

Antiphospholipid antibodies occur in association with a variety of conditions, including self-limiting viral and bacterial infections, syphilis, systemic lupus erythematosus (SLE) and other connective tissue diseases, and after coronary artery bypass graft surgery. Depending on the antibody specificity, they may be detected as lupus anticoagulant, as anticardiolipin antibodies or as anti-$\beta 2$ glycoprotein I antibodies. Antiphospholipid antibodies often appear only transiently, or at low titre, in the circulation. Thus, in the absence of SLE or another disease associated with a high risk of thrombosis, their prognostic significance is considered uncertain, unless there is a history of thrombosis or adverse pregnancy outcome, in which case the patient is defined as having primary antiphospholipid syndrome.

Treatment of thrombosis in antiphospholipid syndrome usually requires indefinite anticoagulation with warfarin. Aspirin may be added if recurrent arterial thromboses have occurred despite therapeutic-range warfarin treatment. A sub-group of patients exist, however, in whom thromboses have only occurred in a pro-thrombotic setting, for example in conditions associated with elevated oestrogen levels. For these patients, a clinical decision is reached with regard to the merits of anticoagulation, with its risk of haemorrhage, as opposed to avoidance of pro-coagulant situations.

In pregnancy, a combination of aspirin and low-molecular-weight heparin is effective in reducing the risk of miscarriage, thrombosis and pre-eclampsia.

Answer 5

    (a) Rheumatoid arthritis   *(1 mark)*

    (b) (i)   Sjögren's syndrome, scleromalacia
         (ii) Rheumatoid nodules, vasculitic rash
         (iii) Pleural effusion, rheumatoid nodules, pulmonary fibrosis
         (iv) Pericarditis, pericardial effusions
         (v) Chronic renal failure secondary to amyloid and drugs, eg gold salts   *(5 marks)*

(c) Patient education on the disease and complications
Physiotherapy, occupational therapy and orthotist
DMARDs, e.g. methotrexate, sulfasalazine,
leflunomide, gold
Intra-articular corticosteroid injections
Analgesia, e.g. paracetamol, NSAIDS
Anti-TNFα agents, e.g. infliximab, etanercept,
adalimumab
Anti-B-Cell agents, e.g. rituximab
Community support
Surgical intervention   *(4 marks)*

Comment

Rheumatoid arthritis is a common, chronic inflammatory arthropathy, which has multiple extra-articular manifestations. It has an autoimmune basis, with important genetic factors. It is associated with HLA-DR1 and -DR4, and has increased prevalence amongst certain racial groups, particularly some of the Native Indian tribes of North America. Environmental factors, including viral and bacterial infections, have also been implicated.

Immune markers for the disease include the classical rheumatoid factor, which is an IgM directed against IgG, and antinuclear factor (ANF). Both of these markers occur in several other rheumatological disorders and their exact role in pathogenesis remains unclear. High titres of the rheumatoid factor has prognostic implications and signifies increased likelihood of extra-articular manifestations.

Recent evidence suggests that rheumatoid arthritis should be treated aggressively as soon as possible after diagnosis. Irreversible damage occurs early but the disease process is more responsive to treatment at this stage. Early intervention thus improves outcome and reduces progression. The aim of treatment is to suppress synovitis and to prevent the development of erosions. DMARDs are usually effective alone but anti-TNFα or anti-B-cell agents may be added in severe disease. Corticosteroids are used sparingly because of the adverse consequences of long-term use. All

DMARDs have multiple side-effects, including renal impairment and bone marrow suppression, and their use should be supervised and reviewed regularly by a rheumatologist. Patients also benefit from education, physiotherapy, occupational therapy and community support to minimise disability. The incidence of cardiovascular disease is considerably increased in comparison to the general population and risk factors should be modified where possible.

Answer 6

(a) Osteoarthritis of the right knee joint   *(1 mark)*

(b) Periarticular sclerosis
Loss of the joint space
Osteophyte formation
Periarticular cysts
Soft tissue swelling
Healed fracture of the distal femur   *(5 marks)*

(c) Dietary advice, weight loss
Analgesia
Physiotherapy
Walking aids as appropriate
Consider surgical arthroplasty   *(4 marks)*

Comment

Osteoarthritis is the commonest of all arthritides, its prevalence increasing with age, affecting 70%–75% of the over 75s population. It is a disorder of the synovial joints, particularly affecting the weight-bearing joints of the lower limbs. Pathologically it is characterised by loss of the articular cartilage and bony overgrowth. It has a multi-factorial aetiology, the exact causes remaining unclear. Factors which predispose to development of the arthritis include:

- Familial tendency
- Hereditary disorders, eg Ehlers–Danlos syndrome, the mucopolysaccharidoses

CHAPTER 11 – ANSWERS

- Concomitant bone disease – Paget's bone disease, Perthe's disease, osteopetrosis, congenital dislocation of the hip (CDH)
- Repetitive occupational trauma, eg professional football players, professional ballet dancers

Answer 7

(a) Systemic lupus erythematosus (SLE)   *(1 mark)*

(b) Anti-double-stranded DNA (anti-dsDNA) antibody
Anti-smooth muscle (anti-SM) antibody
Anti-cardiolipin antibody
Anti-Ro antibody
Anti-La antibody
Anti-U1 ribonuclear protein (anti-UIRNP) antibody
(3 marks)

(c) (i)   Butterfly (malar) rash, photosensitive rash, discoid lupus
(ii) Raynaud's phenomenon, vasculitic rash, venous thrombosis
(iii) Glomerulonephritis, chronic renal failure
(iv) Psychoses, seizures, peripheral neuropathy, cranial nerve palsies
(v) Coombs-positive haemolytic anaemia, thrombocytopenia
(vi) Myopathy, non-erosive arthropathy   *(6 marks)*

Comments

Systemic lupus erythematosus (SLE) is the commonest of the collagen vascular disorders, with a prevalence of 40–65:100 000. It is nine times more common in women and is particularly prevalent amongst black women in the United States and the Caribbean. The peak incidence is between 20 and 40 years. It is a multisystem disorder, but most commonly presents with musculoskeletal and cutaneous manifestations and symptoms. The skin changes may be part of the multisystem disorder or may be almost totally confined to the skin, known as discoid lupus. Several of the auto-antibodies which occur have been linked to specific syndromes within the disease. Anti-dsDNA has been linked to the development of nephritis, anti-Ro and anti-La to the photosensitivity syndrome, and the anti-cardiolipin antibody (the lupus anticoagulant) to the syndrome of recurrent miscarriage, thrombosis and thrombocytopenia. The mainstay of treatment remains maintenance therapy with oral steroids, with the use of immunosuppressants, such as azathioprine and cyclophosphamide, being reserved for acute exacerbations of the disease.

Answer 8

(a) Raynaud's phenomenon   *(1 mark)*

(b) Calcinosis
   Raynaud's phenomenon
   Oesophageal dysmotility
   Sclerodactyly
   Telangiectasia
   The syndrome is now termed limited cutaneous
   systemic sclerosis   *(4 marks)*

(c) Educate the patient and family about the disease and
   prognosis
   Raynaud's – treatment and prophylaxis
   Skin care
   Immunosuppression
   Nutritional support – may require gastrostomy feeding
   if dysphagia is severe
   Treatment of specific complications – pulmonary
   fibrosis, pulmonary hypertension chronic renal
   impairment   *(5 marks)*

Comment

Progressive systemic sclerosis (previously called scleroderma) is a multi-system connective tissue disease that principally presents with skin changes and Raynaud's phenomenon. It is three to four times more common in women and its peak incidence is between 30 and 60 years. It is now subdivided into limited and diffuse cutaneous disease.

The limited disease, previously termed the CREST syndrome, is the more common. The associated Raynaud's phenomenon – whereby the digits become painful and progress through several colour stages, ie white to cyanosed to red, on exposure to the cold – requires both prophylaxis and treatment. Avoidance of cold exposure and protection against the cold with heated gloves and socks is the main prophylaxis. Calcium-channel blockers, ACEIs and 5-HT2 inhibitors, are used in long-term therapy, with a prostacyclin infusion reserved for the more acute cases.

The diffuse disease affects the lungs, heart, bowels and kidneys most commonly. Pulmonary fibrosis causes increasing respiratory failure, leading to pulmonary hypertension. Unlike the limited disease, the entire bowel may be affected by dysmotility problems, and as the disease progresses this will require increasing nutritional support. Cardiac manifestations include cardiomyopathy, myocarditis and pericardial effusions. Several immunosuppressants are used in the treatment of the disease, but as yet none has been shown to influence the prognosis.

Answer 9

(a) Gout *(1 mark)*

(b) Serum uric acid
X-ray of the left foot
Examine joint aspirate under polarised light microscopy for negatively birefringent crystals
(3 marks)

(c) Risk factors:
      Increased purine turnover – leukaemia, psoriasis
      Increased purine synthesis – Lesch–Nyhan syndrome
      Alcohol excess
      Drugs – thiazide and loop diuretics, low dose aspirin
      Toxins – lead
    Drug therapy:
      NSAIDs, eg indomethacin – renal impairment
      Colchicine – diarrhoea
      Allopurinol – worsens acute gouty episode

(6 marks)

Comment

Gout is the commonest of the crystal deposition disorders, and is caused by abnormal uric acid metabolism, leading to the deposition of sodium urate in the joints, soft tissues and renal tract. It presents in middle age and is more common in men, and the upper social classes. In most patients the disease is idiopathic, although there are several predisposing conditions.

Hyperuricaemia is a marker for the disease, but is ten times more common than symptomatic gout. The disease leads to an erosive arthropathy, commonly effecting the distal interphalangeal joints of the fingers and the interphalangeal joints of the toes. It should always be considered in the differential diagnosis of an acute monoarthritis.

The treatment of gout is divided for the acute and chronic disease. In an acute attack, NSAIDs or colchicine is used. Long-term therapy is aimed at reducing the risk factors, treating any predisposing conditions and the use of allopurinol. Allopurinol should not be given within four to six weeks of an acute episode as it may precipitate another acute episode.

Answer 10

(a) Polymyalgia rheumatica
   Giant cell arteritis   (*2 marks*)

(b) Rheumatoid arthritis
   Multiple myeloma   (*2 marks*)

(c) (i)   Temporal artery biopsy   (*2 marks*)
   (ii) High-dose steroids (50–60 mg od)   (*1 mark*)
   (iii) Angina, temporal headaches, stroke
         Sudden blindness
         Jaw claudication   (*3 marks*)

Comment

Polymyalgia rheumatica is an idiopathic disorder which presents between the ages of 50 and 70. It classically produces an ESR of more than 100, and clinically is associated with early morning stiffness of the shoulder and pelvic girdle muscle, which improves slowly with exertion. There is no definitive investigation for this disorder and anyone with suspected disease should be started on a trial of oral steroids. These may be slowly reduced according to the clinical response and the reduction in the ESR. Most patients are able to stop the steroids within two to three years of the diagnosis being made, but relapses are quite common.

Temporal arteritis may be regarded as the opposite end of a spectrum with polymyalgia. It is caused by a giant cell arteritis, which can affect facial, cerebral, cardiac and mesenteric arteries, and thus produces a varied group of presenting features, including jaw claudication with talking or eating, angina and sudden blindness due to involvement of the retinal artery. It is therefore essential to start steroid therapy in any suspected cases, and attempts should be made to obtain histological confirmation by temporal artery biopsy. There is a 48-hour window between starting the steroids and obtaining the biopsy, before the steroids affect the histological changes and make the biopsy valueless.

Answer 11

(a) Wegener's granulomatosis
Classical triad: upper and lower respiratory tract, and
renal involvement   *(4 marks)*

(b) Rheumatoid arthritis
Polyarteritis nodosa
Streptococcal infection
Drug allergy
Mixed essential cryoglobulinaemia   *(2 marks)*

(c) FBC, clotting screen, ESR
c-ANCA, and other autoantibodies
CXR
Bronchoscopy and biopsy
Renal ultrasound scan
Renal biopsy
Cyclophosphamide is the drug of choice   *(4 marks)*

Comment

Wegener's granulomatosis is a small vessel vasculitis associated
with the formation of granulomata. It remains an idiopathic
disease, but the relatively recent identification of the
autoantibody c-ANCA, and more precisely the antiproteinase 3
antibodies, has led to an improvement in both the understanding
of the pathogenesis and treatment of the disorder. These
antibodies are present in 80%–85% of cases and are immune
markers for the disease. They are also used to follow the success of
therapy and to monitor disease activity. Clinically the disorder is
characterised by the classical triad above, but also produces
multiple systemic features, including malaise, fever, myalgia and
polyarthritis. Skin and eye involvement are common, and the
disease may also affect the central and peripheral nervous
systems, causing hypothalamic–pituitary dysfunction and
mononeuritis multiplex.

Treatment of the disease initially includes cyclophosphamide and steroids; these may be reduced slowly, depending on the response. Other cytotoxics such as azathioprine may be used instead of cyclophosphamide.

Answer 12

(a) Osteoporosis   *(1 mark)*

(b) (i) Poor dietary calcium intake during adolescence
         Premature menopause (as in this case)
         Lack of weight-bearing exercise
         Prolonged amenorrhoea – long distance runners,
         anorexia nervosa   *(3 marks)*
    (ii) Medications:
         Analgesia
         Cyclical bisphosphonates
         Hormone replacement therapy
         Calcitonin   *(3 marks)*

(c) Advice to her daughter should include:
    Regular weight-bearing exercise
    Maintain a good diet with adequate calcium intake
    Avoid alcohol excess and smoking   *(3 marks)*

Comment

Osteoporosis is a common metabolic bone disorder that principally occurs in postmenopausal women. Pathologically it is characterised by a decrease in bone mass without a change in the bone's cellular composition.

Peak bone mass occurs in the early 20s, and its subsequent rate of loss is dependent on genetic and environmental factors, as well as intercurrent illnesses. It is therefore important that during the growth period of childhood and adolescence, individuals maintain adequate nutrition and particularly 'load' their diet with calcium. All other risk factors should also be addressed. Post-menopausal women should be offered hormone replacement therapy (HRT), although at present it is unclear as to how long this should continue. Long-term use is associated with an increased incidence of breast cancer. Women suffering a premature menopause, either due to autoimmune disease or surgical removal of the ovaries, are particularly at risk, not only of developing osteoporosis but also ischaemic heart disease.

The diagnosis is confirmed by X-ray findings and DEXA scan, which may also be used in assessing a patient's risk of developing the disease. Confirmed cases or those presenting with fractures of a long bone or vertebrae should receive a bisphosphonate or one of the newer therapies such as strontium or PTH. Bisphosphonates inhibit osteoclastic bone resorption, and are particularly useful in vertebral bone disease. Acute cases require analgesia and may benefit from the use of calcitonin, which has been shown to improve outcome and has some analgesic effect.

Answer 13

(a) Increased bone turnover with associated remodelling and defective mineralisation *(2 marks)*

(b) Radiographs of the right hip, pelvis and lumbar spine
Serum calcium, phosphate and alkaline phosphatase
Urinary hydroxyproline *(3 marks)*

(c) Complications:
Bone pain
Vertebral collapse and resultant paraplegia
'High output' cardiac failure
Deafness
Osteosarcoma
Therapeutic management:
Adequate analgesia
Bedrest
Bisphosphonates, calcitonin or mithramycin
(5 marks)

Comment

Paget's disease of the bone is a common metabolic bone disorder, which occurs after the age of 40. Its prevalence increases with age, particularly in women. The disease is idiopathic, but latest theories propose a viral agent, due to the discovery of viral-like inclusions seen within the osteoclasts. Several viruses have been studied including RSV, measles and canine distemper virus.

Clinically it presents with pain and bony deformity, classically causing anterior bowing of the tibia and enlargement of the skull. The bones may feel warm due to increased vascularity, and pathological fractures may occur, particularly in the pelvis and the vertebrae, where subsequent collapse can lead to spinal cord compression. The progression to osteosarcoma is rare, occurring in only 1% of cases. Investigations will reveal a normal calcium and phosphate with an elevated alkaline phosphatase, which reflects the increased osteoblastic activity. A raised calcium should alert the physician to the possibility of concurrent malignancy, hyperparathyroidism or prolonged immobility.

Patients should be treated with bisphosphonates, which decrease the excessive bone turnover. Calcitonin is used for bony pain and in the postoperative period of patients undergoing joint arthroplasty, where it reduces bleeding. Rarely, mithramicin is also used.

Answer 14

(a) HLA-B27
Reiter's syndrome, psoriasis, inflammatory bowel disease *(3 marks)*

(b) Ankylosis of the vertebrae with syndesmophyte formation – 'bamboo spine'
Calcification of the spinous ligaments
Sacro-ileitis *(3 marks)*

(c) (i) Anterior uveitis
(ii) Conduction system fibrosis
(iii) Upper zone pulmonary fibrosis
(iv) Atlanto-axial subluxation with resulting cord
compression and tetraplegia *(4 marks)*

Comment

Ankylosing spondylitis is a progressive inflammatory disorder, which is particularly prevalent in young men. It causes severe back pain which is classically worse in the morning and improves with exercise. Progression of the disease leads to a gross reduction in the range of movement of the cervical and lumbar spine, causing the patient to develop a marked kyphosis. This, in association with the loss of the lumbar lordosis, produces the classical 'question mark' posture. Extra-articular manifestations are common and are as follows:

- Pulmonary: apical fibrosis; although commonly quoted this is in fact relatively rare
- Cardiac: conduction system fibrosis, leading to varying degrees of heart block. An ascending aortitis occurs with associated aortic valve regurgitation; pericarditis and cardiomyopathy may also occur
- Eyes: anterior uveitis, this occurs in 25%–30% of cases
- Renal: secondary amyloidosis may occur causing chronic renal failure

Treatment should include NSAIDs for analgesia and more importantly a physiotherapy programme, which retards the spinal deformity. In patients where NSAIDs are ineffective, sulphasalazine is used, but the use of other immunosuppressants has failed to influence the long-term prognosis.

Answer 15

(a) Reiter's syndrome
Urethritis, conjunctivitis and arthritis   *(2 marks)*

(b) *Chlamydia* spp
Campylobacter jejuni
Shigella
Yersinia   *(3 marks)*

(c) Investigations:
    FBC, blood cultures
    HLA typing
    Urethral swabs for chlamydia and other STDs
    Syphilis serology
    Aspiration of knee joint for microbiological review
    Consider HIV test with pretest counselling
Therapeutic management:
    Appropriate antibiotics, eg ciprofloxacin
    Bedrest; non-weight-bearing on affected leg
    Counselling and education about the disease
    Contact tracing of any sexual contacts   *(5 marks)*

Comment

Reiter's syndrome is a characterised by the triad of conjunctivitis, urethritis and a reactive arthritis. The associated arthritis is aseptic and usually affects a single joint, particularly of the lower limb. The disease is strongly associated with HLA B27, and is usually precipitated by a gastrointestinal or urogenital infection. The syndrome has several other acute manifestations, including anterior uveitis, circinate balanitis, Achilles' tendonitis, plantar fasciitis and keratoderma blenorrhagicum. Clinically the disease may have one of three courses: an acute illness with complete resolution; a prolonged single episode, which lasts over six months and requires immunosuppressants; and a recurring, episodic disorder, which may be due to reactivation with a new infection or solely due to the original illness. It is important that the patient is made aware of the possibility of recurrence.

12

ANSWERS

Psychiatry

Answer 1

    (a) Atypical antipsychotic   *(1 mark)*

    (b) (i) Agranulocytosis
         (ii) Registration of patient, prescriber and pharmacist
            onto a clozapine patient monitoring service
            Full blood count with white cell differential before
            starting drug, every week for 18 weeks then every
            fortnight. May be reduced to no less than once
            every four weeks after one year of treatment if
            stable   *(4 marks)*

    (c) Failure to adhere to treatment
         Alcohol misuse
         Cannabis use
         Incorrect tablet strength dispensed
         Incorrect diagnosis (bipolar disorder with manic
         psychotic episodes rather than schizophrenia)
                                 (5 marks)

Comment

Table: Classification of antipsychotic drugs

Class	Drug	Side-effect profile		
		Extrapyramidal*	Antimuscarinic**	Sedative
Phenothiazine derivatives				
Group 1	Chlorpromazine, Levomepromazine, Promazine	++	+	+++
Group 2	Pericyazine, Pipotiazine	+	+++	+
Group 3	Fluphenazine, Perphenazine, Prochlorperazine, Trifluoperazine	+++	+	+
Non-phenothiazine classical antipsychotics				
	Benperidol, Haloperidol, Pimozide, Flupentixol, Zuclopenthixol, Sulpiride	+++	+	+
Atypical antipsychotics				
	Amisulpride, Aripiprazole, Olanzapine, Quetiapine, Risperidone, Sertindole, Zotepine	• Generally better-tolerated than older drugs • Weight gain and glucose intolerance, particularly with olanzapine and clozapine • Extrapyramidal side-effects usually occasional, mild and transient • Hyperprolactinaemia less common than with older drugs		
	Clozapine	• As for other atypical antipsychotics, plus: • Agranulocytosis • Myocarditis and cardiomyopathy • Gastrointestinal obstruction		

* **Extrapyramidal side-effects** comprise Parkinsonian signs and symptoms, dystonia, akathisia (restlessness, which may be difficult to differentiate from the effects of continuing psychosis) and tardive dyskinesia.

** **Antimuscarinic side-effects** include dry mouth, blurred vision, constipation and urinary retention.

Answer 2

(a) **C** – have you ever felt you should **C**ut down on your drinking?

A – have people **A**nnoyed you by criticising your drinking?

G – have you ever felt bad or **G**uilty about your drinking?

E – have you ever had to take a drink first thing in the morning to steady your nerve or get rid of a hangover? (**E**ye opener) *(4 marks)*

(b) MCV

LFTs and gamma glutamyl transferase *(2 marks)*

(c) Obtain a full history from the patient and wife – separately if required

Screening tests

Patient must accept there is a problem before further help can be given

Acute withdrawal – diazepam and psychological support

Long-term support:

Alcohol abuse self help groups, eg Alcoholics Anonymous, deterrent drugs

Psychiatric help may be required *(4 marks)*

Comment

Alcohol abusers or problem drinkers are an extremely heterogeneous group of individuals, crossing all social and economic barriers. It is estimated that approximately 1:20 adults in the UK are problem drinkers, with 25% of inpatients estimated to have alcohol-related problems. Despite the recent changes recommended by the Department of Health, the medical community still regards the 'safe' limits for alcohol consumption to be 14 units/week for a woman and 21 units/week for a man (where one unit is equal to a single measure of spirits, a glass of wine or a half pint of beer).

Problem drinking causes psychological, physical and social problems, which are dose related. Physical and psychological dependence will cause withdrawal symptoms within 12 to 24 hours of abstinence. The physical symptoms include palpitations, tremor, sweating, retching, vomiting and seizures.

Several syndromes arise due to the direct effects of the alcohol or its withdrawal:

- Delirium tremens – this presents on alcohol withdrawal with an altered level of consciousness, confusion, agitation and tremor In extreme forms there may be associated aural and visual hallucination and paranoid delusions
- Korsakov's syndrome – characterised by short-term memory loss and confabulation
- Wernicke's encephalopathy – this is associated with confusion, nystagmus and VIth nerve palsy

The most difficult part of treatment of the problem drinker is the acceptance that there is a problem, and abstinence. Once this has been achieved, physical withdrawal may be attempted, usually aided by the use of diazepam (chlormethiazole is still used in some hospitals, but it remains an expensive and relatively poor drug for this situation). Nutritional deficiencies, particularly vitamin B complex, should be corrected, parenterally if necessary.

Answer 3

(a) Elderly, male
Long suicide note
Recent bereavement   (3 marks)

(b) Method of attempt
Precautions against being discovered
Seeking help prior to or after the attempt
Planning of the attempt   *(3 marks)*

(c) Management
Initial therapy:
   Endotracheal intubation, IV access
   Blood tests:
      FBC, U&Es, glucose, LFTs, clotting, paracetamol
      and salicylate levels (serum should be saved for
      other drug levels, eg tricyclic antidepressants)
      Activated charcoal via nasogastric tube
      Specific treatment directed against the tablets he
      has taken
Psychiatric therapy:
   Must be admitted as this was a serious suicide attempt
   Antidepressants
   Bereavement counselling   *(4 marks)*

Comment

Non-fatal deliberate self-harm or parasuicide has dramatically
increased in incidence over the last century, now leading to
almost 100 000 acute admissions per year in the UK. The
commonest method, accounting for 90% of cases, is self-
poisoning, principally with paracetamol, aspirin, minor
tranquillizers and antidepressants.

Self-poisoning is more prevalent amongst young women
particularly in lower social classes, although recent trends have
shown increased rates amongst young men.

Important factors to consider in the history of a patient presenting
with non-fatal deliberate self-harm are:

- Family or personal history of previous suicide attempts
- Family or personal history of psychiatric illness
- Personal relationship problems
- Employment stress or unemployment

- Recent bereavement
- Social isolation
- Financial problems
- Concurrent serious or chronic illness

It is estimated that 20%–25% of self-poisoners will make further attempts. This is increased if there is evidence of alcohol or drug abuse, psychiatric illness, social isolation and unemployment.

Answer 4

(a) Anorexia nervosa
Body weight reduced by 10%–15% of expected or previous weight
Self-induced weight loss by avoidance of fattening foods   *(3 marks)*

(b) Body mass index (BMI) = weight in kilos/(height in metres)^2
= 30 / 1.60^2
= 30/2.56
= 11.72 (normal range = 20–26)   *(3 marks)*

(c) Investigations:
FBC and MCV
U&Es
Albumin
Calcium, phosphate and magnesium
Vitamin B12, folate and ferritin
TFTs
FSH/LH
Anti-endomysial antibody
Management:
Confirm the diagnosis by history and investigation
Address underlying psychological or social problems
In mild cases – regular follow-up and dietary advice
More severe cases – admit to specialist unit;
nutritional support, psychiatric therapy   *(4 marks)*

Comment

The major eating disorders are a product of modern Western society and have become prevalent only in the last 20–30 years. They are made up of the two extremes in body form, anorexia and bulimia nervosa at one end of the spectrum, and obesity with associated psychological problems at the other. Anorexia nervosa is a complex disorder that usually occurs in adolescence and early adulthood, and is particularly prevalent in girls of this age. Bulimia is recognised as a variant of anorexia, with self-induced vomiting associated with intractable overeating. Both are considered to be primarily psychiatric disorders, with psychological, emotional and environmental causative factors. The diagnostic criteria for anorexia nervosa were defined by the ICD-10:

- Body weight maintained at 15% or more below that expected, or in prepubertal patients, failure to make expected weight gain during the growth period
- The weight loss is self-induced by avoidance of fattening foods and is associated with at least one of the following – self-induced vomiting or purging, excessive exercise, the use of appetite suppressants or diuretics
- The dread of fatness is viewed as an intrusive, overvalued idea, and there is self-imposition of a low weight threshold. This is accompanied by amenorrhoea in the female and loss of libido and impotence in the male. There is also delayed or arrested puberty in prepubertal patients

Answer 5

(a) (i) Opiate overdose
Immediate management:
IV access protection of the airway
IV naloxone   *(3 marks)*
(ii) Pinpoint pupils will confirm the diagnosis
(1 mark)

(b) Intravenous – known as 'mainlining'
Smoking/inhalation – known as 'chasing the dragon'
(2 marks)

(c) (i)   Neurological – agitation, paresthesia and dilated pupils
(ii) Psychological – depression, craving
(iii) Gastrointestinal – diarrhoea, vomiting, abdominal cramps
(iv) Dermatological – sweating, 'goose bumps'
(4 marks)

Comment

Opiates remain one of the most commonly abused group of drugs, mainly in the form of heroin. It may be injected, smoked or even taken in tablet form. Psychological and physical dependence are common in regular use, but unlike many drugs tolerance means that addicts must increase their intake to maintain the same level of effect.

Withdrawal, commonly known as 'cold turkey' because of the associated shivering and goose bumps, is extremely unpleasant, but is rarely life threatening. Both physical and psychological symptoms are prominent. Medically supervised withdrawal involves replacement of the heroin with methadone (which itself may become the focus of addiction), and slow reduction in the dose. This period should involve a specialist unit, to provide community, social and psychological support.

It must be remembered that various drugs have been abused throughout history, and what is regarded as illicit to one culture remains acceptable to another. Although opiates, hallucinogenics, stimulants and sedatives remain illegal in the Western world, many more people suffer illness and death each year through alcohol- and nicotine-related disease. Health-care professionals must remain impartial and resist being judgemental.

Answer 6

(a) Reactive depression – bereavement reaction
Loss of interest in person and environment
Loss of appetite, weight loss
Insomnia, early morning waking   *(3 marks)*

(b) Psychotherapy – including bereavement counselling
Cognitive therapy
In severe cases – electroconvulsive therapy (ECT)
                                          (2 marks)

(c) Tricyclic antidepressants, eg amitriptyline –
anticholinergic side-effects, eg dry mouth
Selective Seratonin Re-uptake Inhibitors (SSRIs),
e.g. fluoxetine, paroxetine – hyponatraemia
Serotonin and Noradrenaline Re-uptake Inhibitors
(SNRIs), e.g. Venlaflaxine, duloxetine nausea and
vomiting, dizziness, somnolence
MAOIs, e.g. Phenelzine – causes a hypertensive
crisis with amines   *(5 marks)*

Comment

Depression may be divided into primary or endogenous and
secondary or reactive. Clinically patients may present with features
of both, and this often makes the division academic. The table
below shows the features of each.

	Primary	Secondary
Identifiable precipitating factor	No	Yes
Premorbid personality	Stable	Often predisposing personality trait
Environmental influences	Unresponsive to environmental influences	Fluctuates according to environmental factors

The somatic features are common to both, eg anorexia, diurnal mood, early morning waking, insomnia.

Therapy is divided into pharmacological and psychological treatment. In mild to moderate depression patients often do as well with psychoanalysis and counselling as with drug therapy. In more serious cases, however, the patients often require both forms of therapy and in very severe cases may also require ECT.

Answer 7

(a) Auditory hallucination
Delusional perception   (2 marks)

(b) Premorbid – unemployment, poor home environment
Presenting – insidious onset, multiple first rank symptoms   (4 marks)

(c) Medical therapy:
    Acute – antipsychotics, eg chlorpromazine
    Chronic – depot injection of a phenothiazine
    (usually fortnightly)
    Psychiatric therapy:
    Psychiatrists and community psychiatric nurses
    Multidisciplinary team:
    Psychologists, counsellors and family education
    and support   (4 marks)

Comment

Schizophrenia is a common psychotic illness, with a prevalence of 2–4 per 1000 of the population. Both environmental and genetic factors have been implicated in its aetiology, but the exact mechanisms remain unclear. Several abnormalities of neurotransmitters within the central nervous system have been identified, including excess dopaminergic activity and abnormal monoamine oxidase levels.

Schneider, in the early part of the twentieth century, coined the phrase 'first rank symptoms'. Exhibition of these symptoms at presentation in the absence of other organic causes, particularly drugs, is highly specific to the diagnosis. These are:

- Auditory hallucination
- Thought withdrawal, insertion or interruption
- Thought broadcasting
- Delusional perception
- Somatic passivity
- External control of emotions

Prognosis is variable, and depends on several factors. A relatively good prognosis can be expected when the illness develops acutely, has a clear precipitating factor, and the patient's premorbid personality and environment were stable.

Answer 8

(a) Mania
Manic depressive or bipolar affective disorder

(3 marks)

(b) Increased energy and activity
Lack of sleep
Grandiose ideas and delusions of grandeur
Increased libido *(3 marks)*

(c) Haloperidol – parkinsonism, confusion, sedation, neuroleptic malignant syndrome
Lithium – nephrogenic diabetes insipidus, confusion, coma, tremor, vomiting and diarrhoea *(4 marks)*

Comment

Mania is an abnormal state characterised by an elevation of mood, increased energy and activity and ideas of self-importance. It presents with a spectrum of symptoms, ranging from a mild to moderate disorder, termed hypomania, to a florid psychotic state. Patients may fluctuate between symptoms of mania and episodes of depression, known as a bipolar affective disorder. This is more common than isolated mania, and is more prevalent in women than men. More unusually, patients may exhibit symptoms of both depression and mania at the same time, termed mixed affective disorder. Clinically, patients have rapid or forced speech, with 'flight of ideas'. They also express grandiose ideas, and occasionally have delusions of grandeur. Acutely, patients require admission to a psychiatric unit, and antipsychotics. Lithium is also used in the treatment of acute mania and in long-term maintenance therapy. It has a narrow therapeutic window and levels must be carefully monitored. Toxicity initially causes blurred vision, diarrhoea, nausea and vomiting, progressing to confusion, seizures and coma. Other side-effects include hypothyroidism, hypokalaemia and rarely, chronic renal impairment.

Answer 9

(a) Dyssocial, psychopathic or sociopathic *(2 marks)*

(b) Personality disorder is an exaggeration of personality traits, which lead to suffering by the individual or others
Examples – paranoid, schizoid, emotionally unstable
(5 marks)

(c) Genetic factors
Developmental factors:
  Environmental factors
  Constitutional disorders
Psychological factors *(3 marks)*

Comment

Personality disorder is a complex concept in which there is an exaggeration of the normal personality traits. The ICD-10 classified the disorder into the following subtypes:

- Anxious or avoidant
- Dependent
- Dyssocial or psychopathic
- Emotionally unstable
- Histrionic
- Obsessive compulsive or anankastic
- Paranoid
- Schizoid

The importance of various factors that influence the development of these abnormal personalities remains unclear. It is known from work with monozygotic twins that genetic factors do play a role, as do constitutional factors. Normal personality is formed principally through psychodynamic and psychological influences during childhood. Thus, in predisposed individuals, it is believed that abnormal influences cause the development of these abnormal personality disorders.

Therapy is based on individual and group psychotherapy, with behavioural modification and social skills training. However, in dyssocial disorders, individuals are often violent and they require treatment in specialist, secure units with various psychotherapeutic and behavioural approaches employed.

Answer 10

(a) Obsessive – compulsive disorder   *(2 marks)*

(b) Neurosis – is an inappropriate emotional or behavioural response to a perceived stressor
Examples – anxiety states, phobic conditions   *(4 marks)*

(c) Treatment principally involves behavioural psychotherapy, ie response prevention; modelling and confrontation
Medications, eg tricyclic antidepressants   *(4 marks)*

Comment

Unlike the psychotic patient, the neurotic never loses contact with reality, and has normal mental functioning. Obsessive–compulsive disorders arise due to obsessional, unwanted thoughts, which the patient cannot resist even though they realise they are wrong. The repetitive rituals or actions they perform as a result of these thoughts are known as compulsions. If these compulsions are resisted the patient often becomes depressed or anxious.

Therapy for these patients is principally based on behavioural psychotherapy. Response prevention is where the patient is encouraged to initiate self-restraint when faced with compulsive actions, eg in the case above, the man would be asked to delay washing his hands, and would have someone observe and encourage him whilst he did so. Initially the observer is the therapist or nurse, but with time a family member may take over this role.

Modelling is the process whereby the therapist demonstrates (models) to the patient that their compulsive thoughts are not based on rational ideas. This may be combined with confrontation, where the patient is repeatedly exposed to a situation which would normally initiate their compulsive behaviour. The idea being that with time the anxiety is greatly reduced, so the stimulus is lessened. Some patients benefit from antidepressants, which gives some credence to the theory that these disorders arise due to abnormal 5HT and dopamine activity. The prognosis is usually good, but is worsened with insidious onset or chronic presentations.

Care of the Elderly

Answer 1

(a) If the diagnosis is correct, potentially curative treatment may be possible.

Even if curative treatment is not possible, surgical resection and/or chemotherapy may reduce the risk of acute bowel obstruction and transfusion-dependent anaemia.

However, potentially curative treatment cannot be offered without a firm diagnosis, which cannot be achieved without investigation.

He may lack capacity to give informed consent to investigation and/or treatment.

After discussion with carers it may be felt inappropriate to offer potentially curative treatment (for instance, because colostomy care would be impossible, or because he would be unable to comply with requirements for safe provision of chemotherapy or radiotherapy).

If it is felt inappropriate to offer potentially curative treatment, investigation itself is unethical.

Palliative treatment would then represent the most ethical choice.

At every stage, he should be assumed to have the capacity to make decisions about his medical care unless it is shown that he lacks capacity.

If he is deemed to have capacity to make a decision, it should be respected, even if it seems eccentric or self-destructive.

When it is deemed that he lacks capacity to make his own decisions, every action taken should be in his best interests. *(6 marks)*

(b) He should be able to comprehend the information relevant to giving or denying consent, particularly:

- the possible diagnosis and its prognosis with and without treatment
- the nature of the investigation, its risks and potential benefits.

He should be able to retain the information for long enough to use it.
He should be able to use the information and weigh it to arrive at a decision.
He should be able to communicate his decision.

(4 marks)

Comment

Mental incapacity is a frequently occurring problem in elderly medicine. Decisions regarding investigation, treatment, withdrawal of treatment and resuscitation are commonplace. So too are issues such as housing, modification of the home, rehousing and finance. The process of making ethical decisions frequently involves consultation with a large number of individuals. Family, friends and neighbours often act as formal or informal carers, and local authorities, private organisations, social workers and general practitioners may be involved in the organisation of care. One or more individuals may have been appointed by a patient to act on their behalf under a Lasting Power of Attorney. The Court of Protection may also have appointed deputies and/or independent advocates to represent a patient's interests. Finally, a patient may have made an advance directive, prior to losing the capacity to take decisions, regarding their future treatment.

Five principles are acknowledged in law as being fundamental to every decision, medical or otherwise, regarding a patient with mental incapacity. First, each patient should be assumed to have the capacity to make a decision until proven otherwise. Second, a patient should be offered every practicable assistance to reach their own decision before it is concluded that he or she lacks the capacity to do so. Third, an apparently unwise decision should not be taken as evidence that a patient is incapable of taking that decision. Fourth, every decision taken or act performed on behalf of a patient who lacks capacity should be in his or her best interests. Lastly, the basic rights and freedoms of the patient should be respected and any decision taken or act performed should be the least restrictive option with regard to these rights and freedoms.

On a practical level, it is important to recognise that mental incapacity should be assessed on a decision-by-decision basis and not applied as a label to an individual. Furthermore, many conditions result in either transient or fluctuating cognitive ability. It may thus be appropriate to delay a decision until such time as the patient is able to take it for him- or herself.

If the cognitive defect is permanent, non-urgent decisions with important implications should be delayed until adequate consultation with all relevant individuals has taken place. This is not necessary, however, where urgent decisions are required for the treatment of acutely life-threatening conditions.

Answer 2

(a) (i) Colorectal carcinoma
  (ii) The differential in an elderly patient such as this would include
   • Diverticular disease
   • Ischaemic colitis
   • Infective colitis – including viral and bacterial enteritis
   • Inflammatory bowel disease – although this is very rare to present de novo at this age
   • Iatrogenic – constipation with overflow (although these would rarely be associated with blood and mucous)
   • Other causes would be suggested by the history and examination   *(4 marks)*

(b) Palpable mass, either abdominal or on digital rectal
examination
Pallor
Hepatomegaly
Distant lymphadenopathy   *(2 marks)*

(c) Routine investigations would include
- Bloods – FBC, U+Es, RBG, LFTs, Calcium, ESR.
- Stool culture – to include *C.difficile* toxin (if indicated)
- Flexible sigmoidoscopy followed by colonscopy; CT
  colonography may also be used
- Radiology – CXR, CT abdomen

Management of a malignant cause should be guided by
the patient's wishes and their co-morbidities. Where
appropriate, surgical and oncological opinion should
be sought.   *(4 marks)*

Comment

Change in bowel habit is a commonly occurring symptom,
particularly in the elderly. A change to less frequent passage of
harder stools is not alarming, unless it is accompanied by other,
more worrying, symptoms. However, a persistent (more than six
weeks' duration) change in bowel habit, characterised by either an
increased frequency of bowel motions, or a change to passing
looser stools, or by both abnormalities, should result in urgent
investigation. Under current guidelines, young patients with
change in bowel habit should not be referred for urgent
investigation unless they have other features suggestive of
colorectal carcinoma, such as weight loss, anaemia or rectal
bleeding (in the absence of anal symptoms). In elderly patients, the
risk of colorectal carcinoma is much greater, so a change in bowel
habit alone is sufficient.

Answer 3

(a) Faecal impaction with overflow, probably due to a
combination of immobility, opiate analgesia and
inadequate diet and water intake   *(2 marks)*

(b) Disimpact the faecal mass with the examining finger and with enemas and suppositories

If this is unsuccessful, manual evacuation under anaesthesia may be necessary

Once rectum clear, prescribe laxative, eg docusate sodium

Try to reduce opiate use but not at the expense of encouraging mobility

Encourage oral intake

Check thyroid function tests and serum Ca^{2+} *(4 marks)*

(c) Trauma to internal and external sphincters and/or pudendal nerve, eg:
    Obstetric trauma
    Surgery for haemorrhoids or anal fissures
    Non-iatrogenic accidental injury

Impaired motor or sensory neurological pathways, eg:
    Stroke
    Dementia
    Multiple sclerosis
    Cauda equina syndrome
    Alcoholic peripheral neuropathy
    Diabetic neuropathy
    Myasthenia gravis

Impaired external anal sphincter and/or puborectalis function, eg:
    Muscular dystrophy
    Myotonic dystrophy
    Senile degeneration
    Rectal prolapse

Inadequate rectal volume, eg:
    Torrential diarrhoea
    Rectal fibrosis secondary to:
        inflammation in ulcerative colitis
        radiation
        ischaemia

Functional disorders, eg:
    Dyssynergic defaecation
    Inadequate access to toilets (in institutionalised elderly)   *(4 marks)*

Comment

Faecal incontinence is a rare presentation in the well elderly but is more common in those living in nursing homes and those with severe cognitive impairment. It usually results from a combination of factors, principally severe physical disability including neurological disability and cognitive impairment. These are often exacerbated by iatrogenic causes e.g. opiate based analgesics and anti-muscarinics. Patients require regular toileting to avoid constipation and overflow diarrhoea, as well as regular fluids and foods. Laxatives may be required to aid the movement of faeces along the ageing bowel but in turn should be used judiciously as they are one of the commonest causes of incontinence in the elderly.

Answer 4

(a) Dementia – probably vascular dementia (previously known as multi-infarct disease) *(1 mark)*

(b)
Name	Name of the prime minister
Address for recall	Name of the monarch
Date of birth	Date of the WW1 or WW2
Place	Recognition of two people
Year	Count backwards from 20 to 1

(5 marks)

(c) Social history:
   Housing
   Mobility ± aids
   Continence/toilet facilities
   ADLs
   Present carers and how they are coping
   Present social services input
Multi-disciplinary team:
   Physiotherapist, occupational therapist
   Dietician
   Continence advisor
   District nurse liaison
   Dementia support team
   Social worker
Consider day care, luncheon clubs and respite admissions to help carers *(4 marks)*

Comment

Dementia is defined as 'a syndrome of the loss of intellectual function and memory, which leads to the breakdown of normal daily functioning, whilst the level of consciousness remains unaffected'.

The prevalence increases exponentially after the age of 65, affecting 3%–4% of those aged 65, increasing to 20%–25% at 80.

Seventy-five per cent of cases are caused by primary degenerative dementia, which includes senile dementia of the Alzheimer's type (SDAT), and vascular dementia (MID). Although these are two separate clinical and pathological entities, many patients have a combination of the two.

Classical Alzheimer's disease occurs in the under 65s, and is characterised pathologically by the presence of neurofibrillary tangles in the cerebral cortex. It has a relatively malignant course, with rapid deterioration of mental abilities and premature death; in SDAT, which occurs in the over 65s, there is a more benign course.

Vascular disease classically gives a stepwise progressive loss in intellectual function, the steps reflecting multiple cerebrovascular events that vary in their size and clinical effect. The patients often have multiple risk factors for atherosclerotic disease.

Although the other causes of dementia account for only 15%–25% of cases, they are important to exclude, as they can on occasion be reversible:

- Infective – AIDS dementia complex (progressive multifocal leukoencephalopathy, cerebral toxoplasmosis and cryptococcus infection), tertiary syphilis, Creutzfeldt–Jakob disease
- Primary neurological disease – Lewy body dementia, Pick's disease, multiple sclerosis, Parkinson's disease, progressive supranuclear palsy
- Metabolic – chronic dialysis, chronic hypoglycaemic episodes, vitamin B12 deficiency

- Malignancy – primary and secondary tumours
- Endocrine disease – hypothyroidism, Addison's disease, acromegaly
- Drugs – chronic use of barbiturates, lithium, cimetidine, anticholinergics
- Toxins – alcohol, heavy metals, eg lead, mercury

Answer 5

(a) Right basal pneumonia
Diabetic precoma
Atrial fibrillation – may be secondary to myocardial infarction
Possible collapse secondary to MI, stroke or arrhythmia, with associated aspiration pneumonia   *(1 mark)*

(b) Haematological:
FBC, U&Es, glucose, Troponin, blood cultures
Non-haematological:
ECG, CXR, MSU, ABGs
Consider CT head scan   *(5 marks)*

(c) Management:
IV access
Broad-spectrum antibiotics
IV insulin sliding scale
Treatment of fast AF – digoxin or amiodarone
NGT – consider enteral feeding
Sub-cutaneous heparin   *(4 marks)*

Comment

The acute confusional state or delirium is a common presentation in the elderly. As in this case, the elderly patient often presents with multiple pathologies, and it may be difficult to decide the primary disorder and the secondary sequelae. It is therefore important to consider all of the possible diagnoses and 'cover' the patient for the most serious or life threatening. In the care of the elderly patient, it should be remembered that it is the patient's premorbid health that is the main determinant of outcome and not their chronological age. In all cases a sense of perspective must be maintained, and one must always try to be appropriate in one's treatment.

Causes of acute confusional states include:

- Sepsis – commonly due to chest and urinary tract infections. However, many patients present with non-specific symptoms and deteriorate rapidly. Therefore, antibiotics are often given empirically in the sick elderly patient, not only to cover primary sepsis but also the near inevitable secondary sepsis that occurs in this group of patients
- Neurological – TIAs, stroke, subdural haematoma, epilepsy, intracerebral tumours – benign and malignant
- Metabolic – hyper- and hypoglycaemia, hyponatraemia, hypercalcaemia, uraemia
- Drugs – sedatives, diuretics, neuroleptics, antiepileptics, digoxin
- Endocrine – Addison's disease, hypothyroidism
- Others – paraneoplastic syndrome, GI bleeds, hypoxia, hypercapnia

Answer 6

(a) Simple falls, eg poor mobility
Postural hypotension secondary to medications
Anaemia secondary to aspirin
Arrhythmias – IHD, medications, electrolyte derangement
Brainstem TIAs   *(3 marks)*

(b) FBC, U&Es, digoxin level
Lying/standing blood pressure
24-hour ambulatory ECG monitoring
Consider OGD and EEG   *(3 marks)*

(c) ACEI – first dose hypotension, dry cough, worsening renal impairment
Loop diuretics – postural hypotension, hyponatraemia, hypokalaemia
Digoxin – arrhythmia, nausea and vomiting
Aspirin – peptic ulceration *(4 marks)*

Comment

Falls are a common cause of morbidity and are markers of mortality in the elderly, with 50% of those sustaining a fractured neck of femur dying within one year. Common causes include:

- 'Simple' falls (these have no identifiable causes, and may be due to a combination of environmental and constitutional factors)
- Environmental (loose carpets, unstable furniture, uneven/slippery floors)
- Cardiovascular (tachy/bradyarrhythmia; complete heart block, significant aortic stenosis, silent myocardial ischaemia)
- Neurological (TIAs, stroke, epilepsy, Parkinson's disease, vertebrobasilar insufficiency, carotid hypersensitivity)
- Drugs (antihypertensives, anti-dysrhythmics, oral hypoglycaemics, psychotropics)
- Toxins (alcohol)
- Other causes of postural hypotension (low output heart failure, autonomic dysfunction)

Constitutional factors which increase the likelihood of falling include visual and auditory impairment, dementia, muscular weakness, nutritional deficiency, chronic systemic disease, and age-related changes in postural and gait reflexes.

Answer 7

(a) Untreated urinary tract infection
Worsening dementia
Poor mobility
Medications, eg diuretics *(3 marks)*

(b)   U&Es, glucose
      MSU
      Urine cytology
      USS of bladder, ureters and kidneys
      Flexible cystoscopy   *(3 marks)*

(c)   Simple measures:
          Incontinence pads ensure regular toileting and easy
          access to toilet facilities
          Review medications – dose and frequency
          Treat underlying infections; atrophic vaginitis
      Others:
          Anticholinergics, eg oxybutynin
          Surgical correction of urological or gynaecological
          abnormalities
          Long-term catheterisation   *(4 marks)*

Comment

Urinary incontinence is a common reason for admission in the elderly, and is deemed to be one of the four 'geriatric giants', with immobility, confusion and falls. Chronic or recurring incontinence may be divided into four categories:

- **Stress** – this is characterised by the loss of small volumes of urine, with increases in the intra-abdominal pressure, eg with laughing or coughing. It is principally caused by bladder outflow tract and pelvic floor weakness, and usually requires surgical correction
- **Urge** – this is caused by detrusor muscle instability, which may be associated with local urogenital disease – cystitis, urethritis or tumours; neurological conditions – dementia, CVA, spinal cord compression
- **Overflow** – this is usually associated with mechanical pressures on the bladder outflow tract causing urinary retention, with associated secondary overflow, eg obstruction – prostatic enlargement, urethral stricture, tumours; neuropathic bladder – diabetes, multiple sclerosis, spinal cord compression

- **Functional** – this is due to an inability to reach the toilet through physical or cognitive impairment, eg confusional states, arthritis, depression, medications

Reversible causes should be addressed, but if incontinence continues then conservative measures should be considered, as listed above.

Answer 8

(a) Premorbid health – malnutrition, pre-existing systemic disease
Pathological fall – MI, arrhythmia, stroke
Operative complications, significant blood loss, prolonged anaesthesia
Postoperative complications – sepsis, confusion, anaemia, depression   *(3 marks)*

(b) FBC, U&Es, glucose, TFTs, calcium
Pre- and postoperative ECGS
CXR
Lying and standing blood pressure
Consider – 24-hour tape, CT head scan   *(3 marks)*

(c) Check all the above investigations treating any reversible factors, eg UTI
Ensure adequate analgesia whilst trying to avoid polypharmacy
Multi-disciplinary input:
    Physiotherapy, occupational therapy
    Social workers
Continue to monitor progress, and liaise with orthopaedic surgeons   *(4 marks)*

Comment

The speed by which patients recover from surgery depends on preoperative, operative and postoperative complications. Elderly patients with increased co-morbidity and polypharmacy often take longer than younger patients and therefore may require more intense preoperative planning to maximise their health and prevent postoperative complications.

Fit, elderly patients do well with surgical intervention and should not be excluded on the basis of age. In orthopaedics the use of spinal anaesthesia and more efficient internal fixation, which can be inserted rapidly, have decreased postoperative mortality.
In all patients who fall, sustaining a fracture, 'sinister' causes must be excluded, including IHD, arrhythmia, stroke, sepsis and increasing confusion.

Answer 9

(a) Hypothermia
Environmental – malnutrition, poor heating
Hypothyroidism
Sepsis
Stroke
Drug overdose   *(3 marks)*

(b) FBC, U&Es, glucose, amylase, Troponin, TFTs, blood cultures
CXR
ECG
MSU
ABGs   *(3 marks)*

(c) IV access
Protect the airways
IV fluids (cautiously)
IV antibiotics
Treat the underlying cause
Warm the patient slowly – blankets, warmed fluids
Subcutaneous heparin (unless contraindicated)
                    (4 marks)

Comment
Hypothermia is defined as a core temperature below 35°C. Any patient presenting with an axillary or oral temperature below 35°C

should have a rectal temperature performed with a low reading thermometer. The elderly are particularly prone to hypothermic events due to environmental and systemic factors, and loss of thermoregulatory control mechanisms. It usually arises as a result of another major pathology, eg stroke, MI, falls or sepsis, although it may occur in isolation, particularly in the winter months. Whatever the cause, it generally has a poor prognosis in this age group, and carries a 50% mortality once core temperature falls to below 32°C. Treatment should be directed at the underlying cause, and the slow warming of the patient, the aim being to increase the core temperature at a rate of 0.5°C per hour. Warmed intravenous fluids should be given cautiously, as they may precipitate pulmonary oedema. Even when sepsis is not the principal cause of presentation, it is almost invariable in the unconscious, elderly patient, and it is recommended that they are given empirical broad-spectrum antibiotics. The elderly are also at risk from thromboembolic disease and should be given prophylactic subcutaneous heparin.

Answer 10

(a) Symptoms of the underlying disease, ie prostatism, retention, incontinence
Gastrointestinal – nausea, vomiting, constipation, appetite, weight loss
Pain – site, character, radiation, relieving and exacerbating factors
Insomnia
Mood *(3 marks)*

(b) Anti-androgenics – cyproterone
Analgesics – simple, combinations, opiates
Steroids
Anti-emetics
Night sedation
Laxatives and enemas *(3 marks)*

(c)   Treatment of underlying disease – cyproterone, local
radiotherapy, TURP
Radiotherapy to bony metastases
Palliation of specific symptoms, eg pain, depression,
nausea, insomnia
Specialist nurse and medical team involvement
Family support
Consider hospice care   *(4 marks)*

Comment

Palliative care is an integral part of the treatment of the dying
patient. With improvements in our understanding of the
molecular and anatomical basis of disease, and the therapeutic
options available, it has become a major speciality in its own
right. The aims of therapy move away from curing the patient to
alleviating distress, and allowing the terminal period, which may
vary from days to months, to be as pleasant and dignified as
possible. The major symptom categories which must be
addressed, are:

- **Gastrointestinal** – appetite (may be improved by use of oral
  steroids); nausea and vomiting; constipation (commonly due to
  opiate analgesia, therefore usually foreseeable; patients started
  on opiates should receive regular laxatives, and may require
  enemas and even manual evacuation); dysphagia (may be due to
  the underlying disease, or candidiasis); weight loss
- **Pain** – as in any patient there is only one rule of analgesia and
  that is to 'be appropriate'. Until the patient is comfortable or
  pain free, one should consider all forms of analgesia. Simple –
  paracetamol, NSAIDs; mechanical therapy – massage,
  reflexology, TENS; combination – coproxamol, codydramol,
  aspav (aspirin and papaveretum); opiates – slow release
  morphine sulphate, morphine elixir, subcutaneous infusion;
  others – spinal and nerve blocks
- **Sleep** – sedation and appropriate analgesia usually allow the
  patient to sleep. However, it must be remembered that some
  people are quite happy with two to three hours of sleep per night
  and should not be over-sedated for the staff's convenience!

- **Mood/psyche** – depression, denial, anger and exhaustion are all common symptoms, which are all exacerbated by poor palliation of the physical symptoms listed above. Counselling should be appropriate

Steroids often help with low mood and poor appetite, but antidepressants and psychiatric intervention may be needed.

Essay Writing

14 Structured Outlines

Question 1

A 69-year-old male smoker presents with a four-month history of a productive cough, episodic haemoptysis and exertional dyspnoea. Discuss the differential diagnosis, and your management of the most likely cause.

Plan

Differential diagnosis:

    Bronchogenic carcinoma

    Tuberculosis

    Bronchiectasis

    Multiple pulmonary emboli

    Biventricular cardiac failure

    The most likely cause is a bronchogenic carcinoma

History:

    Features of malignancy

Specific:

    Hoarse voice (recurrent laryngeal nerve palsy)

    Visual disturbance – Horner's syndrome

    Paraesthesia and numbness along the ulnar border of the forearm and ulnar two fingers – brachial plexus invasion by Pancoast's tumour

    Ectopic hormone secretion, eg SIADH and parathyroid hormone-like peptide

Non-specific:

    Weight loss

    Anorexia

Constipation
Depression

Examination
General:
Anaemia
Horner's syndrome
Clubbing of the finger nails
Nicotine staining of the hands
Cachexia
Lymphadenopathy – supraclavicular, cervical and axillary
Heptomegaly
Respiratory examinations:
Signs of lobar collapse
Consolidation and pleural effusions
Investigations:
Bloods – FBC, U&Es, LFTs, calcium and phosphate
Sputum – MC+S, AAFBs and cytology
CXR
Bronchoscopy and biopsy
±Aspiration of pleural effusion and pleural biopsy

Therapeutic management is based on investigation results
Options:
Surgical excision ± postoperative radiotherapy
Radiotherapy
Chemotherapy
Palliative care

Question 2

What are the causes of cardiac failure? Discuss the management of a 54-year-old woman who presents with a six-month history of exertional dyspnoea, swollen ankles and three pillow orthopnoea.

Plan

Causes of cardiac failure:

    Acute:

        Myocardial infarction causing left ventricular failure, mitral valve regurgitation and ventricular septal defect

        Arrhythmia

        Bacterial endocarditis

        Pulmonary embolism

        Septicaemia and other causes of multiorgan failure

    Chronic:

        Ischaemic heart disease

        Hypertension

        Idiopathic cardiomyopathy

        Valvular heart disease

        Cor pulmonale

Management:

    This woman's symptoms are suggestive of biventricular cardiac failure

History:

    Specific symptoms of cardiac failure and causative disorders, eg angina

    Risk factors, eg hypertension, diabetes, peripheral vascular disease, smoking, alcohol, obesity and hyperlipidaemia

    Exacerbating factors – β-blockers

Examination:

    Signs of cardiac failure, eg tachycardia, gallop rhythm, raised jugular venous pressure, basal crepitations, peripheral oedema

Other signs:

    Stigmata of hyperlipidaemia, cardiac murmurs, absent peripheral pulses

Investigations:

    Bloods – FBC, U&Es, glucose, lipids, TFTs

    CXR

    ECG

    Echocardiogram

Therapeutic:
  General:
    treat underlying causes, remove exacerbating factors
    address risk factors
  Improve morbidity/mortality:
    ACE inhibitors
    Angiotensin II receptor blockers
    Aldosterone antagonists
    Re-introduce selective β-blocker (carvedilol, bisoprolol or
    metoprolol) carefully when stable
  Improve symptoms:
    Loop diuretics + thiazide (metolazone) if necessary
    Digoxin
  Surgical valve replacement or ventricular aneurysm resection
  Consider biventricular pacing, heart transplant, ventricular
  assist device

Question 3

*Write an essay on the causes and management of
bloody diarrhoea in a 24-year-old woman.*

Plan
Causes:
  Infective:
    Salmonella, Shigella, amoebiasis, *Campylobacter*, HIV-related
    Inflammatory bowel disease, ulcerative colitis, Crohn's disease
    Ischaemic colitis

Management
History:
  Duration of illness
  Diarrhoea – frequency, consistency, colour
  Blood – mixed or separate from stool, quantity
  Associated features – anorexia, weight loss, abdominal pain,
  nausea and vomiting
  Systemic features of IBD

Examination:

    General – clubbing, anaemia, jaundice, cachexia, pyrexia

    Abdominal masses, fistulae

    PR examination – peri-anal disease

Investigation:

    FBC, U&Es, LFTs, ESR

    AXR

    Stool specimen – MC+S, ova, parasites and cysts

    Sigmoidoscopy and biopsy

Therapeutic:

    Based on the cause identified by investigation

Question 4

Discuss the management of a 31-year-old woman who is found unconscious at home after taking an overdose of diazepam and paracetamol tablets.

Plan

Initial management:

    Airway – protect and maintain the airway (will require anaesthetic help)

    Breathing

    Circulation – will need IV access and fluids started

    Cardiac monitor

    Pulse oximetry

    Urinary catheter

    Cardiovascular, respiratory and neurological assessment

Initial investigations:

    FBC, U&Es, glucose, LFTs, clotting, drug levels – paracetamol and salicylates

    CXR

    ECG

    ABGs

Therapeutic management:

    Stomach washout, with protection of airway (not applicable if >1 hour after overdose)

    Activated charcoal via nasogastric tube

Diazepam:
> try flumazenil as a reversing agent for depression of
> consciousness

Paracetamol:
> toxic levels will indicate need for *N*-acetylcysteine infusion
> patient's hepatic and renal function must be closely followed
> with daily INR, LFTs and U&Es

Once patient is medically well enough she will require
psychiatric assessment

Question 5

*Write an essay on the causation and diagnosis of a
first epileptic seizure in a 48-year-old woman. What
therapeutic options could you use to treat her?*

Plan

Causes:
> Primary/idiopathic epilepsy – less likely in this age group
> Secondary:
>> malignant brain tumour
>> metastases – carcinoma of the lung or breast
>> lymphoma
>> intracerebral haemorrhage and thromboembolic stroke
>> subdural haemorrhage
>> intracerebral abscess

Clinical examination:
> Signs of systemic disease
> Papilloedema
> Localising neurological signs

Investigations:
> Bloods:
>> FBC and differential, clotting, ESR, blood cultures (if
>> appropriate)
> CXR
> CT or MRI head scan
> EEG

Therapeutic options:
    Idiopathic:
        anti-epileptics – first line: carbamazepine, sodium valproate
        second-line treatment: phenytoin
        add on therapy – vigabatrin, lamotrigine, gabapentin
    Secondary causes:
        tumours – neurosurgical excision, radiotherapy,
        radiotherapy, chemotherapy
        abscess – neurosurgical incision and drainage with
        postoperative IV antibiotics
        subdural haemorrhage – neurosurgical drainage
        thromboembolic stroke – anticoagulation

Model Essays

Question:

Write an essay on the diagnosis and management of a 56-year-old man who presented to the Emergency Department having vomited two cupfuls (200 ml) of fresh blood a few hours previously.

ANSWER 1 – a comfortable pass

Introduction

Chronic peptic ulceration (gastric and duodenal ulcers), often resulting from *Helicobacter pylori* infection, accounts for approximately half of all cases of upper gastrointestinal haemorrhage. Other causes are bleeding from gastro-oesophageal varices (<5%), reflux oesophagitis (5%), Mallory–Weiss syndrome (5%–10%), acute gastric ulcers and erosions (20%) and, rarely, gastric carcinoma. Other uncommon causes are hereditary telangiectasia, pseudoxanthoma elasticum and blood dyscrasias. Aspirin and other non-steroidal anti-inflammatory agents along with alcohol intake produce bleeding from acute ulcers and these agents make chronic ulcers more likely to bleed.

Initial management

Assessment of the severity of the haemorrhage includes observation of vital signs, with shock defined as pulse >100 beats per minute and systolic blood pressure <100 mmHg. Increasing age and presence of co-morbidities are also important to risk of death This patient has suffered a recent significant though noncatastrophic upper GI haemorrhage and must be admitted to hospital. He would be expected to pass the remaining blood as melaena over the ensuing days. A loss of up to a litre of blood in a previously healthy individual under the age of 60 years is readily compensated haemodynamically. If he shows no evidence of shock and his haemoglobin is >10 g/dl then no immediate resuscitatory measures are required. Bedrest, intravenous access, hourly monitoring of vital signs and urine output with blood grouped and crossmatched are sufficient immediate measures. In addition, an intravenous infusion of omeprazol reduces the risk of rebleeding and the duration of hospital admission. A detailed history and physical examination is carried out along with a peripheral blood profile.

Investigations
The diagnosis may be obvious from the history, eg. a long history of dyspepsia or, more significantly, previous haemorrhage from a peptic ulcer. A history of aspirin or non-steroidal anti-inflammatory drug ingestion would suggest acute ulceration. Signs of chronic liver disease, viz hepato-splenomegaly or stigmata of portal hypertension, would suggest a variceal bleed, but occasionally it may occur from an accompanying peptic ulcer in patients with chronic liver disease.

An upper GI endoscopy (flexible oesophagogastroduodenoscopy) will detect the cause of the haemorrhage in over 80% of cases. If evidence of a recent bleed is seen, ie a visible vessel or an adherent clot, the patient is more likely to rebleed. A low haemoglobin level would suggest chronic blood loss prior to the haematemesis that brought the patient to hospital.

Treatment
Once the cause of the bleeding is identified, treatment measures may be instituted. If an acute bleeding source in a gastric or duodenal ulcer is visualised at endoscopy, the bleeding may be arrested by submucosal injection of 1:10000 solution of adrenaline or by application of a heater probe, multipolar coagulator or mechanical clips. Intravenous omeprazole infusion may be continued for 72 hours to control active bleeding. If evidence of

Helicobacter pylori infection is detected, eradication treatment is prescribed (two antibiotics for one week in addition to continuing proton pump inhibitor). If rebleeding occurs, a further attempt at haemostasis may be made at endoscopy. Surgery may be necessary for further bleeding. After discharge, duodenal ulcers are successfully treated with six weeks of proton pump inhibitor therapy. Patients with gastric ulcers should undergo repeat endoscopy after six weeks of proton pump inhibitor therapy to check that healing has occurred and to exclude malignancy.

Peptic ulceration caused by a gastrin-producing tumour of the pancreas (gastrinoma; Zollinger-Ellison syndrome) is severe and recurrent. Surgical resection of the gastrinoma may not be curative if there are multiple tumours or metastasis has occurred. Acid secretion may be suppressed by high doses of proton pump inhibitors in combination with somatostatin analogues. In those who are non-adherent or nonresponsive to medical therapy, total gastrectomy may be required.

The diagnosis of a malignant gastric ulcer is by endoscopic visualisation and biopsy or barium meal examination. Surgical resection offers the only hope of a cure.

A Mallory–Weiss mucosal tear at the gastro-oesophageal junction is produced by coughing or retching and bleeding usually stops spontaneously; rarely the tear may require suture.

Variceal haemorrhage is unlikely in this patient but would require endoscopic bending of the feeding submucosal veins in the oesophagus. Terlipressin administered as a four-hourly IV bolus reduces the splanchnic blood flow. Octreotide infusion is an alternative. Balloon tamponade with a Sengstaken–Blakemore tube may be necessary if these measures fail. The tube is left in situ for a period of approximately 12 hours followed by re-endoscopy to confirm cessation of bleeding. Variceal bleeding that is uncontrolled by these means necessitates a TIPSS procedure (transjugular intrahepatic porto-systemic shunt) oesophageal transection with ligation of the feeding vessels. Endoscopic surveillance is used to detect and treat recurrent varices with a maintenance dose of oral propranolol to lower the resting pulse rate by 25% which reduces the incidence of rebleeding when the liver disease is well compensated.

General lifestyle measures

Smoking and alcohol consumption along with drugs that provoke mucosal erosions must be avoided. Regular eating habits with adequate rest must be encouraged, along with ways of modifying stresses associated with modern-day living.

Examiner's comments:

- The essay is eminently readable, knowledgeable and concise with appropriate sub-divisions
- The introduction defines the problem and its causes
- Diagnosis is based on the history, examination and investigations with emphasis being rightly placed on the first and the last
- The question is very broad and therefore treatment can only be covered in outline. However, clear guidelines on each treatment modality is given
- The importance of endoscopy for diagnosis and surveillance and its use in treatment for specific lesions is stated
- The need for long-term drug therapy for chronic lesions and the importance of general lifestyle measures is mentioned

ANSWER 2 – an answer showing insufficient knowledge

The diagnosis of this man should involve the following stages: history, examination, investigation, treatment.

The history starts by asking for the mainly formal details, ie name, age, address, GP, date of birth. Next ask for the patient's presenting complaint and record this in the patient's own words. The history of the presenting complaint should involve a review of the relevant system, ie the patient is vomiting blood, so it is necessary to ask about how much blood, the colour of the blood, how long this has been going on for and if he has ever had this before.

Record the patient's past medical history including any operations he has had in the past and illnesses, eg high blood pressure, diabetes, epilepsy, rheumatic fever, jaundice and TB. Ask about the drug history and any allergic responses. Next consider the social history, in which smoking and alcohol are very important. A common cause of haematemesis is excess alcohol consumption producing a Mallory–Weiss tear. Ask about the patient's housing arrangements and, as the patient will undoubtedly have to be admitted, it is important to look into who would take care of the household. Next ask about the family history. Review of systems should encompass respiratory, cardiovascular, gastrointestinal, urogenital and musculo-skeletal systems.

Examination of the patient which follows takes the following sequence: observation, palpation, percussion and auscultation.

Firstly, check for jaundice, anaemia, clubbing, cyanosis, oedema and lymphadenopathy. A full physical examination involving all the systems should follow.

Investigations are the next stage and should include a full blood count, liver function tests, a chest X-ray and blood grouped and cross-matched. A treatment plan is then formulated. The possible causes of this patient's haematemesis are ulcer, mitotic lesion, trauma or alcohol abuse.

Intravenous access should be established and pain relief given. If the patient is feverish it would be necessary to administer antibiotics for a probable infective cause. An exact (definitive) diagnosis may be established when the investigations are to hand.

Examiner's comments:
- Shows a poor understanding of the question and knowledge required to answer it
- The urgent need to establish the diagnosis is not appreciated
- Despite some idea of the possible causes of the bleeding, the candidate has little idea how to identify the bleeding source
- A good deal of time is wasted on an irrelevant history and examination

- There is no mention of treatment of any of the possible causes, nor follow-up

ANSWER 3 – an answer showing insufficient knowledge

The initial stage of the diagnostic procedure is a complete history expressly concentrating on previous episodes, bleeding tendencies, current medication, recent history of vomiting prior to haematemesis, ingestion of alcohol, symptoms of liver disease or peptic ulcer.

Examination would entail: (i) pulse, blood pressure ventilation rate, (ii) signs of anaemia or chronic blood loss, (iii) stigmata of liver disease, (iv) guarding with signs of peritonitis and (v) a rectal examination to exclude rectal bleeding.

Investigations include a full blood count, urea and electrolytes, liver function tests and grouping, cross-matching and saving in case of continued bleeding. Most importantly an endoscopic examination of the oesophagus down to the duodenum to identify a bleeding lesion such as ruptured varices or a Mallory–Weiss tear at the gastro-oesophageal junction or a bleeding ulcer in the stomach or duodenum.

A bleeding vessel can be injected with a sclerosant, such as phenol, or sealed by diathermy or laser. If varices are involved a Sengstaken tube can be passed down and inflated to compress the bleeding source.

Admit and refer to the gastroenterologist; if the cause is traumatic a surgeon may be required.

An important omission is not to prepare for the possibility of shock should the bleeding recur, ie establish IV access and rehydrate with normal saline and/or colloids while blood is being crossmatched.

Examiner's comments:
- Is aware of the urgent nature of the condition and has some idea of the possible causative lesions
- Shows some knowledge of the lesions involved but is insufficient in depth
- No mention of the treatment of the commonest lesion, viz peptic ulcer/erosions
- No mention of follow-up and the management of recurrence

ANSWER 4 – an answer showing insufficient knowledge

The initial management of a patient presenting with haematemesis is to assess his volaemic status. The volume of blood vomited will not be a good indicator of total blood loss, as estimates by the patient will be inaccurate as not all blood will be vomited.

Initial observations of blood pressure, pulse and respiratory rate should be made looking for signs of shock. If this is present the patient should be laid flat, IV access established and an infusion of a plasma expander such as gelofusin started. Even if shock is not present at presentation IV access should be established and blood grouped and saved in case of further bleeding. Observations of BP and pulse should be continued.

Once the patient is stable, a history should be taken. Pertinent questions on the presenting complaint include: time of haematemesis in relation to presentation; the volume and nature of blood in vomit; any associated symptoms; previous episodes and melaena or a history of alcohol abuse, smoking, liver failure or peptic ulcer.

On examination, as well as looking for signs of shock, look for stigmata of chronic liver disease. A PR examination should be performed for evidence of melaena.

Appropriate investigations are a full blood count; a low Hb would indicate chronic bleeding. Bleeding two hours previously is unlikely to produce a drop in Hb as a shift of fluid into the intravascular compartment will not yet have occurred. In addition a slightly raised MCV could indicate a reticulocytosis, further supporting chronic bleeding. A low platelet count could indicate thrombocytopaenia and a bleeding tendency. LFTs for evidence of liver failure; clotting screen for a bleeding tendency; also supports evidence of liver failure. A differential diagnosis would include bleeding oesophageal varices; Mallory–Weiss tear; severe reflux oesophagitis; eroded peptic ulcer; ulcerating gastric carcinoma and trauma.

In distinguishing between these possibilities evidence of liver failure would point towards varices. This is the diagnosis to be differentiated as it is an indication for urgent endoscopy. If this shows varices the bleeding may be controlled by injecting the varices.

If varices are thought to be unlikely the patient should be admitted to an acute bed and kept under observation for signs of shock or further blood loss. If this occurs transfusion should be considered, combined with plasma expanders if necessary. The patient should be kept nil by mouth. Endoscopy should be arranged as soon as possible to make the definitive diagnosis of the cause of bleeding. Many of the causes can now be corrected by endoscopy.

Examiner's comments:
- Too much preoccupation with shock, which kept recurring through the essay
- The urgent nature of the presentation is appreciated
- The need for constant monitoring is appreciated
- The commonest cause for the bleeding, viz peptic ulcer/erosion, is not recognised
- The treatment of variceal bleeding is inadequate
- The treatment of all other causes are not mentioned
- An inadequate knowledge of OGD as a diagnostic and therapeutic tool

CHAPTER 15 – QUESTIONS

ANSWER 5 – an answer showing insufficient knowledge

The patient should be brought into a cubicle and note should be taken of any obvious signs of anaemia or illness. A full history should be taken with particular emphasis on the amount of blood loss and its colour and if the patient experienced pain with the vomiting, viz Mallory–Weiss tear. Had the patient any chest or abdominal pain at other times and whether there was a history of trauma. A poor diet or the intake of spicy food and alcohol intake may predispose to ulcers, along with smoking. A drug history with particular emphasis on the use of pain-killers, viz anti-inflammatory drugs. Any previous episodes should be enquired.

Examination should then follow; first pulse, BP and respiratory rate are measured looking for shock. Then the abdominal system is of principal concern and the following points are of principal interest: the presence or absence of stigmata of chronic liver disease; the presence of anaemia; lymphadenopathy, viz Virchow's node (gastric Ca); any areas of abdominal tenderness; any abdominal masses viz. organomegaly (spleen, liver, kidneys); signs of portal hypertension; a per rectal examination should be undertaken.

Investigations should then follow; blood should be taken looking at full blood count and ESR (for possible anaemia and infection); U&Es, liver function tests and for grouping, saving and cross-matching. A chest X-ray to look for trauma, etc. Eventually the patient will be sent for endoscopy to try to locate the source of the bleeding, the patient being admitted for these investigations. Once these investigations are underway therapeutic options may be taken depending on what is found. Bleeding varices usually require endoscopic intervention as an emergency; they can be injected or compressed. Ulcers that have perforated can be surgically resected.

Examiner's comments:
- A poorly planned attempt with disorganised thoughts
- The urgent nature of the presentation is appreciated and the possible need for resuscitation

- Endoscopy was the last in the sequence of investigations despite realisation that this was essential for a diagnosis of the cause
- There is some knowledge of causative lesions though management of these is at best vague
- There is no mention of the management of peptic ulcer/erosion, the commonest cause of the bleeding

Essay

INFECTIONS

1. Describe how you would investigate a male patient aged 22 with apparent candidiasis infection in the mouth, who had also recently lost weight and become breathless.

2. Discuss the epidemiology, clinical course and possible prevention of Hepatitis B infection.

3. Describe the clinical manifestations of infection with HIV

   What methods are available for: (a) preventing the spread and (b) modifying the course of the disease?

4. What are primary, secondary and tertiary prevention? Giving as an example any communicable disease, describe the prevention strategies for each of the three categories.

5. Compare the causative organisms of bacterial meningitis in the neonate, child and adult. Discuss the management in a 9-year-old girl who is admitted with meningococcal meningitis.

6. What do you understand by the term 'septicaemic shock'? Discuss the common causes and the general principles of your management.

METABOLIC DISEASES

1. Malnutrition complicates many illnesses in an affluent society but is often unrecognized and untreated. Discuss possible reasons why this aspect of disease may be neglected and suggest possible steps that may be taken to prevent diseases associated with nutritional excess.

2. Define obesity. Discuss the relative values of the different methods used to assess the degree of obesity. Describe your regimen for the treatment of simple obesity in a woman of 35 years.

3. Discuss the investigation and management of a 43-year-old man with hypercholesterolaemia.

4. Discuss how you would counsel parents of a child with a newly diagnosed autosomal recessive metabolic disorder of your choice.

   Discuss the prognosis, treatments and the diagnostic tests available.

5. Compare and contrast haemochromatosis with Wilson's disease.

NEUROLOGY

1. Describe the clinical features of migraine and the differential diagnosis from other types of headaches. How would you manage a patient with migraine?

2. Discuss the clinical manifestations of multiple peripheral neuropathy and their relation to the aetiology.

3. Discuss the causes of a facial nerve palsy, and the management of one cause.

4. How would you manage a young woman newly diagnosed with generalized tonic-clonic seizure?

5. A woman of 70 wakes one morning with weakness in her right arm and difficulty with speech. How would you arrive at a diagnosis and what are the probable causes? How would you counsel the patient and her relatives?

6. Discuss how you would investigate and manage a 26-year-old man who presents with an episode of painful, blurred vision and numbness in his hands and feet.

ENDOCRINOLOGY

1. Write an essay on the clinical manifestations and treatment of acromegaly.

2. What conditions may present with the symptom of thirst? What investigations would you carry out on such a patient?

3. Describe the clinical presentation of myxoedema. What investigations would you require to confirm the diagnosis, and how would you treat a 68-year-old woman with this condition?

4. Write an essay on the pathogenesis of primary, secondary and tertiary hypercalcaemia. What are the principles of treatment in each of these conditions?

5. Write an essay on the clinical manifestations of overactivity and underactivity of the adrenal cortex.

6. Discuss the management of uncomplicated diabetes mellitus in the different age groups.

RESPIRATORY MEDICINE

1. Discuss the major differences in history, examination and investigations between the common and atypical pneumonias. Give a brief account of the complications of pneumococcal pneumonia.

2. Describe the management of an acute attack of asthma in a 25-year-old woman.

3. To what can the present rise in the incidence of TB in this country be attributed? What factors may result in this trend being reversed?

4. Write an essay on respiratory failure and its management.

5. Describe the diagnosis, management and clinical associations of pneumothorax.

CARDIOLOGY

1. Discuss the clinical features, diagnosis and management of a 16-year-old girl with infective endocarditis.

2. Write an essay on the complications and management of mitral stenosis.

3. Describe the clinical features of acute myocardial infarction and discuss the immediate management in a 58-year-old man.

4. Discuss the investigation and management of a 51-year-old man with essential hypertension.

5. Give an account of the clinical presentation, differential diagnosis and treatment of acute pericarditis.

6. Describe the causes, clinical features and treatment of congestive cardiac failure.

HAEMATOLOGY

1. Discuss the diagnosis and treatment of iron deficiency anaemia. What factors may slow the response to treatment?

2. Give an account of the symptoms and signs to be found in a patient with pernicious anaemia. How would you treat this patient?

3. Write an essay on the hazards of blood transfusion. What are the features of a transfusion reaction and how would you manage such an event?

4. Give an account of the adult leukaemias. Discuss the investigations required to make a diagnosis and the common treatment modalities used.

5. Discuss the investigation and management of a patient with suspected multiple myeloma.

6. Discuss how you would investigate a patient with haemolytic anaemia; what are the features of chronic haemolytic disease?

DERMATOLOGY

1. What is the 'triple response' of the skin? In what conditions is it produced? How would you investigate and treat a case of urticaria?

2. Discuss the general principles of managing a patient with pruritus.

3. In what disorders and in what ways may hair growth be affected? How would you treat male-pattern baldness?

4. How would you manage a young adult presenting with psoriasis?

5. Write an essay on abnormalities of the nails.

GASTROENTEROLOGY

1. A middle-aged man is brought into the Accident and Emergency department, having vomited a large quantity of blood, and feeling very weak and faint. Describe your immediate management and discuss the investigations required to arrive at a diagnosis.

2. Describe the factors underlying the formation of ascites. Discuss the principles of management when the ascites is due to chronic liver disease.

3. Discuss the investigation and management of a 45-year-old woman presenting with a two-month history of jaundice. (Ultrasound scan shows 'no gall stones present in the gall bladder'.)

4. Describe the clinical features and management of a 28-year-old woman suffering from acute ulcerative colitis.

5. Discuss the clinical presentation, investigations and management of a 24-year-old woman with coeliac disease, listing the differential diagnosis.

6. A 41-year-old man presents with symptoms suggestive of a duodenal ulcer. Discuss your investigation and management.

NEPHROLOGY

1. What are the clinical and biochemical features of 'end-stage' renal failure, and how may it be treated?

2. Discuss the aetiology and management of a young adult with acute glomerulonephritis.

3. Discuss the management of a 21-year-old woman who presents with recurrent urinary tract infections.

4. Discuss the genetics of polycystic kidney disease and outline its management and complications.

5. How would you assess a patient for renal transplantation and how would you prevent post-transplant rejection?

RHEUMATOLOGY AND CONNECTIVE TISSUE DISEASES

1. Discuss the investigations and therapeutic management of a 29-yearold woman who presents with a bilaterally symmetrical polyarthropathy.

2. What impact has immunology made on the diagnosis of rheumatological and connective tissue diseases?

3. A 21-year-old woman presents with an acutely inflamed left knee. Discuss the likely causes and your management.

4. Compare and contrast the systemic vasculitides.

5. Discuss the clinical manifestations and management of a patient with systemic sclerosis.

PSYCHIATRY

1. What are the physical and mental features of severe anorexia nervosa? Discuss the treatment and prognosis.

2. What is a compulsive neurosis? Describe the features, predisposing factors and available treatment measures.

3. A wife reports that her 45-year-old husband is excessively jealous, accusing her of infidelity and threatening to harm her. How would you assess the situation, and advise both the husband and the wife?

4. What are the causes of acute mania and how may they be differentiated and treated?

5. 'Drug abuse is the scourge of the 21st Century'. How does it impinge on the community you live in? Discuss the measures you would adopt as a community physician to counteract this.

6. Write an essay on the social and psychological factors which may lead to attempted suicide in different age groups.

CARE OF THE ELDERLY

1. An 84-year-old woman presents with metastatic carcinoma of the breast. Discuss your investigation and management.

2. A 91-year-old independent man presents with recurrent falls. Discuss your investigations and management.

3. What do you understand by the term 'dementia'? How would you assess and manage a 70-year-old man who is complaining of forgetfulness?

4. An 81-year-old man is determined to go home to his 5th floor flat despite reservations by the hospital medical staff. Discuss how you would ensure that he manages successfully at home.

5. An 80-year-old woman is admitted with mild heart failure, which responds well to treatment. However, after 3 days in hospital she becomes increasingly confused. Describe how you would investigate and manage this development.

APPENDIX A

The Examination in Medicine

Assessment of clinical competence

Medical training encompasses a wide range of complex and varied activities and has evolved to match the diverse abilities required of the practising clinician. Maintaining these skills is essential for the establishment of professional standards of excellence and satisfying public expectation.

Assessment of clinical competence over such a broad field is fraught with difficulty: it has to examine the results of a number of years of study, covering a large syllabus in a uniform, efficient, competent and reliable fashion. It should ensure that candidates who have achieved the required level of proficiency pass, and those who have not should fail. The examination should be seen by students and examiners as being fair.

The perfect examination not only has to accurately assess knowledge and understanding but also evaluate the powers of analysis in problem solving and decision making. In the clinical field to these attributes must be added the candidate's attitude to patients and clinical work and their ability to communicate, as well as their personal and professional development and conduct.

Why examine?

Over the last few decades a number of groups have questioned the need for formal assessment and have proposed continued, faculty-based evaluation in medical education. Nevertheless, the vast majority of medical schools and universities rely on staged examinations, to ensure the acquisition of a minimal knowledge base. Satisfactory performance may be accompanied by graduation, certification and the right to practise. The level of achievement may influence progress and promotion.

Examinations are also valuable for students and teachers to establish personal and departmental standards, and one of the problems of statutory examinations is usually their lack of feedback of the details of a candidate's performance. Internal faculty examinations can be an aid to learning and a means of self-evaluation: this will become of increasing importance with the extension of continued medical education, to help students identify a weakness of personal knowledge and of teaching material. Even the most ardent supporters of continuous assessment cannot deny the stimulus and motivation of an examination, and it does separate good from bad candidates.

What system?
To justify their existence examinations have to be seen to be fair, and linked with both the training and its stated objectives. Traditional medical examinations have been based on the essay, the oral and the clinical. History and examination are central to a doctor–patient relationship, and the clinical has held its ground in undergraduate and postgraduate assessment, although the division between medicine, surgery and other disciplines has often become blurred, the emphasis being on the history and examination rather than the underlying disorder. Short cases in some schools have been replaced or supplemented by Objective Structured Clinical Examinations (OSCEs) to accompany the written part, and orals have been restricted to distinction and borderline candidates.

The essay has come under the greatest scrutiny. Students and examiners have questioned the effectiveness of an essay paper, since the limited number of topics and the possible choice have encouraged students to spot questions and concentrate on only part of the syllabus. The marking of essays is time-consuming and unreliable. There may be variation in an individual examiner's reassessment of papers, as well as between examiners. The variation makes comparison at a national level difficult, and this is further

APPENDIX A

accentuated by what has been described as the deep psychological reluctance of examiners to allocate more than 70% of the total marks allowed for any given essay question. Attempts to modify the essay included modified essay questions (MEQs), which introduce a larger number of questions with a patient vignette, and a variety of sub-sections based on various aspects of diagnosis and treatment. Multiple short answers on a range of topics have also gained favour in some schools. Structured answer questions (SAQs) are a further development of the written assessment, testing problem-solving and decision-making in a structured and objective fashion. They are proving a reliable means of assessing knowledge and understanding in clinical practice.

MCQs also have a wide application in medical assessment, having the potential of covering a wide body of knowledge and, in their extended matching pairs format, introducing reasoned responses rather than item recall. A computerised marking system has eased the examiners' burden in this section. A current trend in the written part of the clinical examination is to include both MCQs and SAQs, the former to determine the candidate's knowledge, and the latter to assess the application of this knowledge by reasoning, interpretation, problem-solving and decision-making.

SAQs
SAQs test the candidate's high-level skills rather than factual recall. They consist of a clinical vignette followed by two to four questions, which may have sub-sections, with an indication of the marks allocated for each correct answer. The choice of scenario is based on common clinical problems pertinent and relevant to the field of study, and covering important concepts and principles relating to the course material. There is no room for trivia, irrelevant or esoteric topics, or interesting rarities.

Clinical information is presented in an ordered fashion, usually describing the history and examination, with or without investigations, of a specific condition. Questions should be clear, unambiguous and requiring the examinee to analyse and make decisions based on the given information. This may involve diagnosis or treatment and may also cover aspects of psychological, social and family history and ethical issues.

Examiners are given a model answer and a marking schedule that has to be closely adhered to. Marking is time-consuming: allotting a single examiner to each question streamlines the process and allows uniformity of marking for a group of candidates. Any allowances made for near-misses will also be generalised. It is common to double mark a number of scripts to check examiners' inter-rater reliability across the whole examination.

Examiners preparing SAQs should form a panel, draw up a list of topics and allocate these topics among the group. The first draft of each question is read out at a group meeting, and comments made on the content, style, the importance, relevance and its educational standard.

The second draft of the questions is tried on a group of students under examination conditions, noting the time taken to complete four to eight questions. The answers are analysed and questions again modified if there are obvious misunderstandings, or unexpected ease or difficulty. Misinterpretation of the stem may lead to an erroneous diagnosis. As the rest of the question is usually based on the stem, a candidate may go off at a tangent in all subsequent answers. The examiners must then make an informed decision in allocating marks for such mishaps, provided the conclusions reached are logical and not far removed from the expected answers. However, in inadequately vetted questions more than one diagnosis may be arrived at from the stem. In such circumstances the onus is firmly on the examiner to accommodate such unanticipated correct responses and mark them fairly.

The completed questions are retained in a question bank. They should be added to each year, attention being given to the choice, number and range of topics. These should match the weighting given to each part of the syllabus.

It may take three to five years to build up an adequate bank, after this time any break in security is of less importance.

APPENDIX A

The stem of a question can often be modified by changing the disease and superficial data, such as the sex, age and the timing of the symptoms. This process eases the generation of further questions and allows some degree of comparison of standards when they are being analysed. Questions should be under continuous reappraisal after each use, to assess their performance and discriminatory value. Marks can be influenced by poor quality of questions, poor knowledge of answers and errors within the marking system.

Each examination requires ten to 12 questions to allow a broad assessment and to produce discriminatory differences between good and unsatisfactory candidates. Each question used should be independent of the others. In qualifying examinations one expects a high pass rate, and a significant number of candidates may achieve distinction level. If this is an entry point to a distinction viva it may be more practical to limit the viva to those within one or two standard errors of the maximum mark obtained.

Essays

MCQs are used routinely in most qualifying and postgraduate examinations. Nevertheless, medicine is not as black and white as MCQs would suggest, and many brighter students are averse to this form of assessment. Similarly, although SAQs allow much wider coverage of the syllabus and more objectivity in the marking systems they also restrict the examiner to black or white rigid marking schemes. The limitations of these features are well known to every clinician who has gone over recent examinations with groups of students.

The essay does test a candidate's ability to collect and quantify material, and assesses their powers of original thought and creativity. It determines the candidate's ability to write clear and legible English, and some schools have felt that these qualities should be retained in their assessment. In spite of the expensive manpower required in marking essay questions, an essay does assess a candidate's depth of knowledge in a specified area and, in preparing for an essay paper, candidates have to acquire detailed knowledge of much of the syllabus.

Revision for the essay paper is linked with revision of the whole course. If a candidate's knowledge base is poor, he or she will rightly fail; but if it is sound, it is essential that their examination technique is good enough to ensure success. The ease of revision is based on previous knowledge and a good filing system which, if disease-based, provides a check list for each condition so that current knowledge can be written and then checked against books and stored material to identify deficiencies.

The candidate is expected to have read around topics and patient problems encountered during the clinical course, gaining information from lectures, reviews, and current papers, as well as text books. This information should be filed in an easily retrievable form, such as notes in the margins of text books, a card system, plenty of lists and clearly written pieces of paper. The internet has become an essential resource and students are advised to link their filing systems to this material. Just downloading un-read and un-classified information, however, is a recipe for disaster – editing and analysis an essential tool in this process. People vary in the amount of information they can remember at any one time. Any deficiency, however, can be easily reversed during revision, provided previous information was well organised and fully understood at the time it was collected.

Examiners at an undergraduate level are keen to pass candidates, to ensure that they can continue with their careers. However, medical examiners have an obligation to ensure that ignorant and potentially dangerous individuals are not let loose on a patient population. At a postgraduate level examiners have to ensure that a candidate has a comprehensive and in-depth knowledge of their subject: gaps are likely to be penalised.

Regardless of the level of the examination, essays on clinical subjects have a similar format. This is based on a disease or a clinical problem and includes questions on the aetiology, pathology, diagnosis, differential diagnoses, complications, assessment, management and treatment. Each question must be read fully and every word noted as they will have been constructed very carefully.

Although the words 'discuss' and a few synonyms imply a certain vagueness, the response must be precise and directed. Having read the question, the answer plan is based on the clinical data required. These will usually correspond to the check list used to revise each disease.

Diagnosis and differential diagnosis are based on only three sources of information; namely, the **history, examination** and **investigation**. If the diagnosis is given, it may require confirmation from the same three sources. Assessment means diagnosis (history, examination, investigation) but adds the dimension of **severity** of the problems encountered. **Management** is assessment plus treatment. Although the term may be loosely used, implying just treatment in some questions, it is worth writing a few sentences on confirmation of diagnosis and severity of the problem being treated. **Treatment** should not be restricted to medicine, as many other problems may require to be sorted out first. Other disciplines that may be involved must be considered, such as nursing, physiotherapy, occupational therapy, and drugs, chemotherapeutic agents and radiotherapy. Radiological intervention forms a major part of treatment in many diseases.

The plan outlining the areas to be covered can be in the answer book or on scrap paper. The plan should take three to six minutes for most essays and allows concentrated thought around the topic. On completion a line is drawn through it to imply to the examiner that there is more to come, and then construct the first few sentences of the introduction. This should imply an understanding of the topic, giving the examiner confidence that the essay is on the right track and, hopefully, is of a good standard.

There is much debate as to whether headings should be underlined and key words highlighted. This debate is more of a problem to the candidate than the examiner, who is more concerned as to whether the script is legible, and demonstrates knowledge and understanding of the question. Illegibility is an inherent problem with some individuals. Examiners go to considerable effort to give candidates the benefit of the doubt but illegibility can never camouflage ignorance, and candidates would be well advised to write at a rate at which the end product is guaranteed readable to the examiner.

Literacy and mastery of prose are more debatable. As much as examiners would wish medical graduates to be able to write skilfully and coherently, marks are predominantly awarded for factual knowledge and understanding of an essay topic. Success is, therefore, based on an appropriate plan and the development of each heading within it.

Medical schools and colleges rarely set regular essays during their courses, even when they use this means of final assessment. It is, therefore, appropriate for students who know they will be examined in this way to undertake preliminary practice. A series of essay questions has, therefore, been added after the SAQs section.

There is a section on planning structural outlines as a preliminary to writing essays, and examples of good and poor answers with examiner's comments. These guidelines may be used in planning and writing essays. The relevant practical information will usually be found in the sectional answers and teaching aids, and essays may be swapped with a working partner or discussion group to act as examiners. Subsequently the plan, development, depth of knowledge, literary style and legibility are discussed. As the exams draw near, the pass standard becomes apparent, and essays can be accurately assessed by peer review.

Whatever examination system is chosen, it must be reliable, valid and discriminatory, and it should not be influenced by the subjective judgement of an examiner. The examination should be about the contents of a paper and not expertise or prior coaching in the chosen system. Nevertheless, it is essential to have prior exposure to the local examination system and be well versed in its technique. This text is intended to provide that exposure and to educate candidates in the techniques of SAQ and essay writing in the hope of easing their passage to qualification.

Self-Assessment SAQ Papers

The Structured Answer Questions in this book are arranged by subject, enabling the reader to focus on individual subject areas and to systematically address any weak areas of knowledge.

However, during revision it is also very valuable to sit authentic test papers. This will help you to become accustomed to working under strictly timed conditions and should also contribute towards making the exam itself a less stressful experience.

The authors have created 12 complete SAQ practice papers, each containing a representative range of topics.

Instructions
- There are 12 questions in each paper, to be answered in two hours.
- You should spend no more than ten minutes on each question.
- The questions have been designed to promote succinct answers.
- Marks available for each section are indicated next to the questions.
- If you are asked for two answers and you give more than two the best two will be marked.

1. 5.4, 2.3, 10.4, 12.3, 7.5, 9.3, 6.4, 1.15, 3.1, 8.7, 4.4, 11.3
2. 5.2, 2.10, 10.3, 13.3, 7.1, 9.4, 6.13, 1.12, 3.7, 8.8, 4.11, 11.5
3. 5.6, 2.7, 9.15, 12.6, 7.6, 9.5, 6.1, 1.11, 3.5, 8.9, 4.2, 11.7
4. 5.7, 2.8, 10.5, 13.7, 7.2, 9.6, 6.2, 1.6, 3.12, 8.10, 4.5, 11.6
5. 5.12, 2.6, 10.10, 13.10, 7.3, 9.1, 6.3, 1.4, 3.8, 6.14, 4.1, 11.2
6. 5.15, 5.9, 10.1, 13.4, 7.7, 9.2, 6.8, 1.3, 3.13, 9.9, 10.7, 11.4
7. 5.10, 3.4, 10.11, 12.7, 7.10, 9.10, 6.7, 1.14, 3.15, 8.6, 10.13, 11.15
8. 5.1, 2.1, 10.13, 12.5, 7.11, 9.14, 6.5, 1.5, 3.2, 8.5, 4.12, 11.8

9. 5.3, 9.6, 10.6, 5.8, 7.12, 9.9, 6.9, 1.10, 3.6, 8.4, 4.14, 11.14
10. 5.13, 2.5, 10.12, 12.4, 9.13, 9.7, 6.15, 1.9, 3.9, 8.2, 10.6, 11.12
11. 5.5, 6.10, 11.9, 12.1, 7.9, 9.11, 6.11, 1.7, 3.16, 8.3, 4.8, 11.11
12. 5.4, 2.9, 10.7, 13.6, 7.8, 9.12, 6.12, 1.13, 3.10, 8.1, 4.10, 11.10